Praise for *Fostering Clinical Success: Using Clinical Narratives for Interprofessional Team Partnerships From Massachusetts General Hospital*

"Over nearly 2 decades, Massachusetts General Hospital has created and institutionalized a narrative culture to enhance patient care. Using the narrative as foundation and turning the lens on the professional self, the approach helps clinicians better understand and articulate their own practice areas and those of their team members. It provides a pathway for professional development and more reflexive clinical practice, decision making, and ethical reasoning."

—Elizabeth J. Clark, PhD, MSW, MPH
President, Start Smart Career Center
Formerly CEO, National Association of Social Workers

"Our narratives about ourselves shape and reveal who we are. *Fostering Clinical Success* shows how narratives shape clinical practice for the better. Filled with real clinical narratives, this book is a manual for how to improve the practice of individual clinicians and how to incorporate narratives into the hospital work culture. It's a great guide for anyone wanting to foster every clinician's best work."

—Jacqueline Hinckley, PhD, CCC-SLP
Author, Narrative-Based Practice in Speech-Language Pathology

"This is a timely and powerful book that provides clinicians, administrators, and educators a road map for transforming our workplace. We know the use of narrative helps practitioners uncover the complexities of practice, the values in tension, and the lived experience of patients. The demand for practitioners who are 'collaboration ready' requires the highest level of critical self-reflection and moral grounding. *Fostering Clinical Success* gives us a structure with explicit strategies for facilitating and transforming our workplace."

—Gail M. Jensen, PhD, PT, FAPTA
Dean, Graduate School and Vice Provost for Learning and Assessment
Faculty Associate, Center for Health Policy and Ethics, Creighton University

"*Fostering Clinical Success* depicts a powerful teaching approach for contemporary healthcare teams that uses a rich array of narratives to help every person on the interprofessional team, including the patient, understand ways of building better communication strategies, better partnerships, better teams, and better team care. The authors use the levels of practice in the MGH clinical model that describe Entry-Level Clinicians, Clinicians, Advanced Clinicians, and Clinical Scholars to help us understand how we think and analyze, given individuals' expertise and where they are in their continuum of practice. The stories are at once both intense and intimate. I highly recommend this book for any health-professions teacher who wants to ensure excellence in the preparation of students for the complexities of today's clinical arena. The authors are world-renowned clinical scholars who have done a beautiful job weaving their own important narratives into what has culminated in a remarkable textbook."

–*Terry Fulmer, PhD, RN, FAAN*
University Distinguished Professor and Dean, Bouve College of Health Sciences
Professor, College of Social Sciences and Humanities
Northeastern University

Fostering Clinical Success

Using Clinical Narratives for Interprofessional Team Partnerships From Massachusetts General

Jeanette Ives Erickson, DNP, RN, NEA-BC, FAAN
Marianne Ditomassi, DNP, RN, MBA
Susan Sabia, BA
Mary Ellin Smith, RN, MS

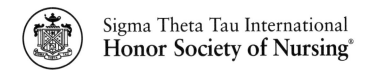

Sigma Theta Tau International
Honor Society of Nursing®

The Honor Society of Nursing, Sigma Theta Tau International (STTI) is a nonprofit organization founded in 1922 whose mission is to support the learning, knowledge, and professional development of nurses committed to making a difference in health worldwide. Members include practicing nurses, instructors, researchers, policymakers, entrepreneurs and others. STTI's 494 chapters are located at 676 institutions of higher education throughout Australia, Botswana, Brazil, Canada, Colombia, Ghana, Hong Kong, Japan, Kenya, Malawi, Mexico, the Netherlands, Pakistan, Portugal, Singapore, South Africa, South Korea, Swaziland, Sweden, Taiwan, Tanzania, United Kingdom, United States, and Wales. More information about STTI can be found online at www.nursingsociety.org.

Sigma Theta Tau International
550 West North Street
Indianapolis, IN, USA 46202

To order additional books, buy in bulk, or order for corporate use, contact Nursing Knowledge International at 888.NKI.4YOU (888.654.4968/US and Canada) or +1.317.634.8171 (outside US and Canada).

To request a review copy for course adoption, e-mail solutions@nursingknowledge.org or call 888.NKI.4YOU (888.654.4968/US and Canada) or +1.317.634.8171 (outside US and Canada).

To request author information, or for speaker or other media requests, contact Marketing, Honor Society of Nursing, Sigma Theta Tau International at 888.634.7575 (US and Canada) or +1.317.634.8171 (outside US and Canada).

ISBN: 9781938835803
EPUB ISBN: 9781938835810
PDF ISBN: 9781938835827
MOBI ISBN: 9781938835834

Library of Congress Cataloging-in-Publication Data

Ives Erickson, Jeanette, author.
  Fostering clinical success : using clinical narratives for interprofessional team partnerships from Massachusetts General / Jeanette Ives Erickson, Marianne Ditomassi, Susan Sabia, Mary Ellin Smith.
     p. ; cm.
  ISBN 978-1-938835-80-3 (print : alk. paper) -- ISBN 978-1-938835-81-0 (epub ISBN) -- ISBN 978-1-938835-82-7 (pdf ISBN) -- ISBN 978-1-938835-83-4 (mobi ISBN)
  I. Ditomassi, Marianne, author. II. Sabia, Susan, author. III. Smith, Mary Ellin, 1954- , author. IV. Title.
  [DNLM: 1. Massachusetts General Hospital. 2. Hospitals, General--Personal Narratives. 3. Patient Care--Personal Narratives. 4. Clinical Competence--Personal Narratives. 5. Nurse-Patient Relations--Personal Narratives. 6. Organizational Culture--Personal Narratives. 7. Physician-Patient Relations--Personal Narratives. WX 28 AM4]
  RA977.5.M4
  362.1109744--dc23

First Printing, 2015

Publisher: Dustin Sullivan   Principal Book Editor: Carla Hall
Acquisitions Editor: Emily Hatch   Development and Project Editor: Jennifer Lynn
Editorial Coordinator: Paula Jeffers   Copy Editor: Charlotte Kughen
Cover Designer: Michael Tanamachi   Proofreader: Todd Lothery
Interior Design/Page Layout: Kim Scott   Indexer: Joy Dean Lee

Dedication

This book is dedicated to the clinicians throughout Massachusetts General Hospital Nursing and Patient Care Services who inspire us to strive for excellence, who make a difference in the lives of our patients and families with their unparalleled compassion and commitment, and who bring the best of themselves and their professions to work every day.

About the Authors

Jeanette Ives Erickson, DNP, RN, NEA-BC, FAAN

Jeanette Ives Erickson is senior vice president for Patient Care and chief nurse at Massachusetts General Hospital (MGH), instructor at Harvard Medical School, and assistant professor at the Massachusetts General Hospital Institute of Health Professions. In her role at MGH, she is responsible for clinical practice, research, education, and global/community health services, serving 5,300 nurses, health professionals, and support staff. She has authored 2 books and several book chapters and articles about her research on the importance of a professional practice environment and other key healthcare initiatives. Ives Erickson has presented globally and consults on multiple issues affecting nurse autonomy, leadership development, collaborative decision-making, and Magnet Hospital designation.

Marianne Ditomassi, DNP, RN, MBA

Marianne Ditomassi is executive director of Patient Care and Magnet Recognition at MGH, which supports the work of the senior vice president for Patient Care and chief nurse, who oversees the operations of nursing, the therapy departments, and social services. Her key areas of accountability include strategic planning, recruitment and retention initiatives, business planning, fundraising, and communications. In addition, Ditomassi is the Magnet Program Director for MGH and successfully coordinated MGH's initial Magnet designation journey in 2003 and subsequent Magnet redesignations in 2008 and 2013.

Susan Sabia, BA

Susan Sabia is the executive editor of *Caring Headlines*, the bi-weekly newsletter for MGH Nursing and Patient Care Services. For each issue, Sabia is accountable for the writing, editing, photography, layout, and design. She studied film-making and creative writing at Ball State University in Muncie, Indiana and Northeastern University in Boston, Massachusetts, and she graduated from University of Massachusetts in Amherst, Massachusetts.

Mary Ellin Smith, RN, MS

Mary Ellin Smith received her bachelor's degree in nursing from Boston College and her master's of science in nursing administration from Boston University. Smith has practiced as a clinical nurse in medicine, critical care, and neuroscience, and she has practiced administratively as a nurse manager and nursing director in medicine and as the director of Professional Practice Development at several large medical centers. She is a professional development manager at MGH in the Institute for Patient Care, where her areas of responsibility include oversight of the clinical recognition program, collaborative governance, and leadership development.

Authors of Clinical Narratives on Interdisciplinary Team Partnerships

Theodora Abbenante, MSHI, RN
Janet Actis, BSN, RN, CPN
Lauren Aloisio, BSN, RN
Susan Barisano, BSN, RN
Julie Berrett-Abebe, MA, MSW, LICSW
Christine Carifio, MS, OTR/L
Heidi Cheerman, DPT, PT, NCS
Meaghan Costello, DPT, PT, NCS
David De La Hoz, BSN, RN
Vanessa Dellheim, DPT, PT
Robert Dorman, PT, DPT, GCS
Kim Erler, MS, OTR/L
Alyssa Evangelista, DPT, PT, OCS, MTC
Katherine Fillo, MPH, RN, RN-BC
Shauna Harris, BSN, RN
Rebecca Santos Inzana, MS, CCC-SLP
Stephen Joyce, AAS, RN
Kristen Kingsley, BSN, RN
Jesse MacKinnon, BSN, RN, OCN
Julie MacPherson-Clements, BA, RRT
Nicole Martinez, BSN, RN
Melissa Mattola-Kiatos, BSBA, RN
Jennifer McAtee, MS, OTR/L, C/NDT
Gloria Mendez-Carcamo, AAS, RRT, RN
Danuza Nunn, MS, CCC-SLP
Brenda Pignone, BSN, RN
Susan Ross, MSW, LICSW
Tessa Rowin, DPT, PT, OCS
Sharon Serinsky, MS, OTR/L
Donna Slicis, MS, APN-BC, CCRN
Janice Tully, BSN, RN, CCM, ACM

Table of Contents

Foreword

Fostering Clinical Success: Using Clinical Narratives for Interprofessional Team Partnerships From Massachusetts General is a joy to read, especially for me as a clinical nurse who went on to become a chief nursing officer, a Magnet® appraiser, and now the chief officer of the American Nurses Credentialing Center. So why is this book a joy? Because it establishes what the clinical profession has intuitively known for years: The power of a story matters.

Patient and family stories have been the safety net and road map for many nurses' clinical treatment plans. But, they lacked credibility because they were just "stories" and not research, evidence, or science. What if stories could be made credible through the systematic approach of research, evidence, and science? Why not fully optimize this way of learning through stories? Why not use stories—or, more accurately, clinical narratives—to enhance the learning environment and clinicians' practice development? The nurses at Massachusetts General Hospital (MGH) did just that, fostering a culture of exceptional practice while they were at it.

Before you start reading this book, let me share a personal story of how I became aware of the clinical narratives work that is so beautifully presented in the pages of this book. In the winter of 2013, I had the honor to be a part of the Magnet® Appraisal Team assigned to Massachusetts General Hospital's third redesignation journey (2003, 2008, and 2013). Boston was enjoying yet another snowstorm as the team arrived. As is generally the case, my journey toward understanding the culture and MGH's Magnet® status began the minute we landed and set off in the taxi ride from the airport to the hotel.

As the taxi driver pulled away from the airport, he asked where I was heading. I shared the address of the hotel. He confirmed the name and said, "It's across the way from Mass General, correct?" I said yes, and the driver asked the nature of my visit and business. I told him my business was nursing, and the conversation blossomed. He shared how a wonderful nurse from MGH had helped his wife when she was gravely ill, had helped his family understand what his wife was going through, and had offered him emotional support. He spoke about the doctors, social worker, and respiratory therapists, but mostly about the nurses.

As he shared his story, it became clear that the respect he had for Mass General came from feelings he had about the "team." As he pulled the taxi up to the hotel entrance, I asked him how his wife was doing. He replied that she had died 6 months earlier from cancer. He said that he was happy, though; his children were grown and were a tremendous support to him, but mostly he was happy his wife was no longer suffering.

He offered great advice on the best place for dinner that evening and then offered a second opinion: "You are a nurse, right? There's no better bunch of nurses than at that hospital." We smiled and said our goodbyes, but his openness about his wife's care stayed with me. It would be just the beginning of the many "stories" the team and I would hear from families, patients, staff, physicians, and community leaders during our Magnet® site visit.

Walking up the driveway to the main entrance, you encounter the many faces of those coming to the facility for care, compassion, and hope. Walking into the main corridor and following the welcome signs to the coffee kiosk, you begin to *feel* the culture of clinical success. An unusual place, right? Not really. This is the hub of the early morning greetings and camaraderie that you see among all the staff—the mixing of friends, colleagues, peers, patients, families, and newcomers. This spirit of the group exudes welcoming care. MGH is a big place, covering many lives and many square miles. The hospital offers the most advanced health-care from some of the most prestigious clinicians in the world to patients and communities it serves, and yet the atmosphere feels welcoming and supportive, like a family.

As the site visit progressed throughout the next 4 days, we traveled through patient care units, specialty services, clinics, old buildings, and new build-ings, all with a similar feeling of teammates working together, appreciating each individual's contribution. On many occasions, I saw student nurses and new graduates during their orientation. I witnessed the willingness of experi-enced nurses to make sure the learning experience was foremost for their new-est colleagues, including new medical residents. It was easy to see and hear the clinical narratives in full operation, fully embraced and enculturated into this organization's fiber.

Our appraisal site visit came to its conclusion. As I had suspected from the first story of teamwork, nursing played a key role in patient and family care. What was most inspiring was that the interprofessional teamwork was so evident and the respect for each other so palpable. This same sense is noted within the pages of *Fostering Clinical Success*—their story, their narratives, their culture.

The interprofessional and interdisciplinary approach that MGH has enculturated through the clinical narrative way of learning is unique and profoundly successful within this world-class healthcare system. I encourage readers to understand that sustained success in this type of journey comes through sustained commitment from leadership—critical for the vision of this type of work. The vision of CNO Jeanette Ives Erickson, DNP, RN, NEA-BC, FAAN, the Nursing and Patient Care Services team, and their many colleagues has brought the clinical narrative to life and fostered their story of clinical success.

As I write these words, Boston is once again under the siege of winter—the Blizzard of 2015. I can't help but think about these team members, their strong culture, and their commitment to the people they serve. They are "Boston Strong." Within these pages you will gain more insight into how they got that way.

With great honor and respect for their work, I offer these humble words of reflection.

Linda Lewis, MSA, BSN, RN, NEA-BC, FACHE
Chief ANCC Officer/EVP
American Nurses Credentialing Center

Introduction

In an environment of rapid change, technological advances, and the ever-growing pressure to deliver care that is efficient and cost effective, some readers may wonder why a book on clinician narratives would be published. The leadership and clinicians throughout Massachusetts General Hospital (MGH) Nursing and Patient Care Services (NPCS) will tell you that the telling and sharing of narratives, or "stories," has been critical in allowing them to understand and address the new healthcare environment and stay true to their essential work—the care of patients and families.

Who This Book Is For

As we reflect on who this book is for, a few recent incidents come to mind to tell us who we think and hope you are:

- A nursing director described a day filled with meetings, reports, and deadlines, as well as a staff nurse's performance appraisal. This nursing director described going through the appraisal with the nurse and then asking the nurse to read her narrative. As the nurse read her narrative, the nursing director explained that she found herself listening to the nurse describing her care of a patient who challenged her and brought her practice to a new level: "I am not sure I would have known about this if she had not shared her narrative with me. Hearing that story and our conversation about it opened so many possibilities in how I can support her and her professional development. I left work that day with so much energy."

- A clinician described writing his narrative as a way to reflect and understand an ethically challenging patient-care situation. He spoke of how often he thought about the patient and all that occurred: "I found that writing down what had happened allowed me to understand my thinking on what I did and why and what I would do differently. Sharing the narrative with my director and clinical specialist brought other resources and supports to assist me and my colleagues in similar situations."

- In a recent program on using narratives to tell stories of error, near misses, or adverse events, a staff nurse described a system issue with a pump that caused the medication to dose to lower than what was prescribed. When asked by the facilitator of the program to read the narrative in front of her very supportive colleagues, the nurse described that being part of the error made her question her practice and filled her with self-recrimination, but being part of this program "has helped me understand, even though everyone told me it was a system issue, that this was not my fault, and my story will help fix this problem."

Who is this book for? For healthcare executives, front-line managers, clinicians from all disciplines, and all those who have watched in awe of a clinician's practice and wondered, "How do they do that? How do they know to do or say that?"

How This Book Is Organized

We have organized this book to reflect our own journey with the narrative.

Chapter 1, "Creating a Narrative Culture," describes the importance of building a foundation of the narrative by building it into the fabric of the organization. This chapter discusses the development of our Clinical Recognition Program (CRP); the themes and criteria for the program were created through the narratives of PCS clinicians in six disciplines.

Chapter 2 defines the first theme of the CRP, "clinician–patient relationship," as the "interpersonal engagement or relational connection between the clinician and the patient and/or family." We share narratives from clinicians across the disciplines, commentary, and reflective questions the narrative raises.

In Chapter 3, the theme "clinical knowledge and decision-making" is defined as the "understanding attained through formal and experiential learning" and is explored through narratives we share from clinicians across the disciplines, through commentaries, and through reflective questions.

In Chapter 4, the theme "teamwork and collaboration" is defined as "through the development of effective relationships with unit-based colleagues and other members of the healthcare team, the best possible outcome is achieved for the patient and family." As with the other chapters, the theme is explored through narratives we share from clinicians across the disciplines, through commentaries, and through reflective questions.

In Chapter 5, "Movement," the theme is specific to occupational therapy and physical therapy. The theme is defined as "through observation, palpitation, and touch the therapist uses knowledge and skill to assess the patients' functional ability" and is explored through narratives, commentaries, and reflective questions.

In Chapter 6, "Strategies to Hardwire a Narrative Culture," we share what has helped us embed the use of narratives across MGH.

Our Goals for This Book

It is our hope that this book allows its readers to do what we all know is so hard to do in this day and age: take time to reflect and engage. We hope that bringing narratives into your practice enables you to understand each other and the practice in new ways. We hope that by listening to others, being present in their story, and then giving the gift of being curious and open to what they are telling you that new knowledge is formed—and that this knowledge creates a safer environment for our patients and an improved professional practice environment for all staff.

Chapter 1
Creating a Narrative Culture

Consider for a moment the following highly impactful and insightful statements:

- "I knew something was wrong."

- "I stayed silent. I knew that she needed time to finish telling me her story rather than the story my questions or comments would lead her toward."

- "I felt a sense of urgency in everything I was doing."

Have you ever been talking with clinicians and heard similar comments and wondered how they knew something was wrong or when and how to intervene? What they saw that others did not? Such questions come not only from curiosity but also from recognizing that you do not know the answer to those questions. And, if you cannot quantify the answer, then how can you possibly evaluate it, teach it, and share it?

It was this frustration that led people in healthcare disciplines—including but not limited to nurses, therapists, and social workers—to seek the answers to these questions using clinical narratives to understand and articulate practice. These stories of clinical practice can be written and shared, and they allow individual clinicians to articulate, reflect, and understand their work. In addition, narratives make visible the clinical excellence and expertise of the clinician and provide an opportunity for shared learning.

Exploring Narratives in the Literature

A clinical narrative is a first person "story" written by a clinician that describes a specific clinical event or situation. Narratives allow clinicians to reflect on who the patient is and how that knowledge informs how clinicians care for patients, make decisions, and collaborate with the members of the healthcare team. Patricia Benner, PhD, RN, FAAN, has written extensively on the use of narratives to articulate skill acquisition in nursing practice (Benner, 1984; Benner, Tanner, & Chesla, 1996) and the clinical wisdom embedded in practice (Benner, Hooper-Kyriakidis, & Stannard, 2011). In her work on educating nurses (Benner, Sutphen, Leonard, & Day, 2010), she used narratives to articulate best practices in teaching and in the student experience of integrating the theory taught in educational programs and the reality of the clinical settings. To understand the informal power of nurses, Paynton (2008) used narratives to identify ways nurses were able to manage systems to advocate for patients. Cathcart and Greenspan (2012, 2013) used narratives to describe skill acquisition in nurse manager practice.

Narratives have given insight into the moral comportment of nurses (Benner, Sutphen, Leonard-Kahn, & Day, 2008) as they care for increasingly complex patients in highly technological environments in the rapidly changing healthcare environment. Narratives are used in multiple disciplines, such as social work (Riessman & Quinney, 2005) and education (Schultz & Ravitch, 2013). In 2009, administrators at the Columbia University College of Physicians and Surgeons inaugurated a program in narrative medicine.

Creating a Narrative Culture

Massachusetts General Hospital (MGH) is a large, tertiary-care, academic medical center deeply rooted in the case study methodology of study and research. Despite the available supporting literature, there were clinicians and leaders who challenged the attention and focus on the narrative as a way to develop reflective practice and professional development. Narratives, many felt, were "too soft" and lacked the rigor found in the case study approach in which data and facts were the focus as the writer walked his or her colleagues through the process of analysis. The MGH senior vice president for patient care and chief nurse who was appointed in 1996 began to educate and influence clinicians' and leadership's understanding of the power of the narrative to articulate and describe the unique role of the clinical disciplines at MGH.

At the time, the department of Nursing and Patient Care Services (NPCS) was fairly new and comprised six disciplines:

- Nursing

- Occupational Therapy

- Physical Therapy

- Respiratory Therapy

- Social Work

- Speech–Language Pathology

The clinicians in these six disciplines primarily worked in silos, with only a broad understanding of what the other disciplines did. The creation of NPCS brought with it some anxiety for the therapists in the therapy departments, as they were joining a service in which they were greatly outnumbered by nursing professionals. They wondered how they could maintain their unique identity and practice.

Through open forums, the senior vice president and chief nurse heard those concerns and began a process in which professionals in each discipline articulated their domain of practice. This process allowed the people in each discipline to reflect on their work and then to share their unique contributions to the care of the patient, the organization, and the team. She then took this work a step further and asked NPCS clinicians to make their domains of practice come alive by telling a narrative that reflected their work as a member of the discipline. She recognized that some clinicians who felt comfortable writing progress notes describing their plan and care of patients and the patients' response to that care might have felt vulnerable in writing a document that described the clinical situation and their thinking and decision-making in the delivery of care to those patients.

NARRATIVES BUILD SKILLED CLINICIANS

Clinicians in MGH's department of Nursing and Patient Care Services have long valued their collaboration with Patricia Benner (1984), whose hallmark book, From Novice to Expert: Excellence and Power in Clinical Nursing Practice, *used narratives to articulate and describe the nurses' changing clinical world as they transitioned from novice to expert. Benner's work built on the Dreyfus Model of Skill Acquisition (1986). Together, the Dreyfus brothers' and Benner's research described that skilled know-how comes not just from knowing what to do—the performance of a task, knowing the policy, or attending a class—but how and when to do it, which occurs in the active engagement with the world. For the healthcare disciplines, this refers to their clinical practice.*

The senior vice president and chief nurse challenged her executive team and nursing directors to create forums and opportunities for clinicians to share their stories. Staff meetings at many units and departments at MGH now include a clinician telling a story about a patient or situation that had meaning for the clinician. Leaders have received coaching on how to use these stories to build reflective practice in their staff. For leaders, this means closely listening to the story and asking unbundling questions that would allow the clinician to move deeper into his or her understanding of the event and, from that, to create opportunity for new learning.

The senior vice president and chief nurse continued her work in creating a narrative culture by setting the expectation that clinicians in NPCS would submit a clinical narrative with their self-evaluation as part of the annual performance review. When staff members challenged this decision, the senior vice president and chief nurse engaged with them on what their experience had been with the existing performance appraisal: Did they believe that the performance appraisal adequately reflected their work and professional development over the past year? The answer was generally no. She then asked staff to reflect on what the performance appraisal experience would be like if they could talk about a situation in the past year that had meaning for them—a situation in which they were at their best or an experience they learned from. Would that story, in addition to the rest of the components of the performance appraisal, demonstrate more about their practice and their ongoing professional needs than the review process already in place? With her leadership, and the leadership of NPCS, the narrative became and continues to be an integral part of every clinician's performance appraisal.

The narratives continued to be woven into the culture of NPCS with their prominent display in the department's bimonthly newsletter, *Caring Headlines*. In the newsletter, a narrative written by a clinician in NPCS is featured, accompanied by a reflective commentary from the senior vice president and chief nurse. Authors of the narratives often receive emails from colleagues, known and unknown, telling them how impressed they were by the practice described in the narrative and asking more questions about it.

MGH NPCS is fortunate to have a robust award and recognition program thanks to its patients and families and benefactors. Every year, clinicians across MGH are nominated for these awards and submit a portfolio, which includes a clinical narrative. Award selection committee members describe that the narrative enables them to see the criteria for the award come to life and informs their decision-making process as they select a recipient.

As narratives became solidly embedded in the culture of MGH, clinicians—who initially might have responded that they did "nothing special" in the care of a patient—told their stories and recognized subtle nuances that they had not identified previously. Through the questioning and curiosity of a colleague or leader, they further explored their interaction with the patient/family, their clinical reasoning, and their work with their peers and members of the healthcare team. For many nurses, therapists, and social workers, narratives allowed them an insight into their actions and thinking that had been missing and made it possible for them to engage in their work more deeply and with greater attention and intention.

The narrative has taught clinicians and leaders at MGH another way of knowing: knowing through the engagement of the clinician in the care of the patient. The narrative allows the reader to enter into the clinician's world—what clinicians are seeing and thinking, and how they are making decisions. The narrative takes the theoretical knowledge of the case study and enriches it with the clinician's experiential knowledge. Through the blend of both sources of knowledge, the story of the patient and the care of that patient and family come into greater focus. This form of knowledge was critical in the development of the MGH NPCS Clinical Recognition Program, in which narratives have enabled us to articulate the themes and criteria of practice for the six disciplines (Nursing, Occupational Therapy, Physical Therapy, Respiratory Therapy, Social Work, and Speech–Language Pathology).

Using Clinical Narratives to Develop an Interdisciplinary Clinical Recognition Program

In 2002, the department of Nursing and Patient Care Services (NPCS) at MGH launched a Clinical Recognition Program (CRP) designed to recognize and celebrate the clinical practice of all direct-care providers. The CRP, the first-of-its-kind interdisciplinary program, needed to meet the professional development needs of clinicians across the healthcare disciplines.

The senior vice president and chief nurse believed that a program to recognize and celebrate the knowledge and skill of direct-care providers was essential to professional development. Not only had clinical staff expressed an interest in such a program, but the senior vice president and chief nurse also felt that an interdisciplinary recognition program would help unite the disciplines and underscore the department's commitment to clinical excellence. In June 1997, she appointed a professional development committee, comprised of representatives from the six NPCS disciplines, to lead the first phase of the program development effort and to develop the framework for a CRP.

Guiding Principles

As a first step, members of the committee articulated a set of principles to guide their work. These principles served several purposes:

- Underscored the importance of the direct provider's role

- Highlighted how experience, collaboration, formal education, and self-reflection promote learning

- Emphasized the importance of recognizing each clinician's contribution to patient care

- Acknowledged the uniqueness of each discipline and the need for inter-disciplinary representation in program development

The principles grounded the group's thinking and ultimately exerted a strong influence on the CRP's framework.

A Conceptual Framework

The committee members then needed to identify a conceptual framework to understand and explicate the practice of the clinicians in NPCS, and their search brought them to the work of Dreyfus and Dreyfus (1986) and Benner (1984). The Dreyfus Model of Skill Acquisition provided a framework for understanding and describing the development of expertise in practice. Benner and her colleagues have worked extensively with the model in clinical settings using the interpretative phenomenology approach of the clinical narrative. Using this approach, the clinical narrative gives the reader insight into the context of the event, including the actions the clinician took and the meaning those actions had.

The committee members put a call out to clinicians across NPCS for their narratives, and it was through reading, discussing, and analyzing those narratives that the committee members were able to identify the themes and criteria for the initial CRP model:

- **Clinician–patient relationship:** The interpersonal engagement or rela-tional connection between the clinician and the patient and/or family.

- **Clinical knowledge and decision-making:** The understanding attained through formal and experiential learning.

- **Teamwork and collaboration:** The development of effective relationships with unit-based colleagues and other members of the healthcare team promotes the best possible outcome for the patient and family.

- **Movement:** Through observation, palpitation, and touch, the therapist uses knowledge and skill to assess the patients' functional ability.

In the introductions to the subsequent chapters, we define these themes that form the framework for the CRP.

Levels of Practice

Returning to the work of the Dreyfus brothers and Benner, the committee members identified four levels of practice that they believed applied to all six disciplines:

- **Entry:** At this level clinicians are learning to apply newly acquired knowledge and skills to a multitude of patient care situations. Entry-level clinicians initially draw on learned facts and rules to organize care and guide practice. As they gain experience, they are increasingly able to recognize the uniqueness of each patient situation and modify care to meet each patient's needs. The Entry-level clinician understands the role of other disciplines and consults with peers in designing a plan of care.

- **Clinician:** At this level clinicians have acquired broad experience in caring for patients and have often developed a sound understanding about the care of a particular patient population. They routinely draw on learned facts and experience as well as an understanding of possible outcomes when designing a plan of care. They have learned to recognize patterns in clinical practice and use this knowledge as they make clinical decisions. They act as resources to colleagues and are strong advocates for patients.

- **Advanced Clinician:** At this level clinicians have typically acquired in-depth knowledge about the care of a particular patient population and an appreciation for the many factors that influence care. In caring for each patient, they constantly consider not just the possibilities—or what could happen—but the probabilities—or what is most likely to happen given the clinical and organizational factors at hand. They routinely consult with and serve as a resource to others and influence practice on their unit/department.

- **Clinical Scholar:** At this level clinicians demonstrate exquisite foresight in planning patient care, are recognized as experts in planning patient care, are recognized as experts in their area of specialization, and are adept at negotiating conflict and collaborating with others. Clinicians at this level are reflective by nature and readily integrate knowledge gained by reflection into their practice. They are able to respond intuitively to patients' needs and engage in clinically sound risk-taking. They are skilled at creative problem-solving, and they routinely lead efforts to strengthen the many organizational systems that support patient care.

By reviewing the narratives, the committee then specified criteria for the levels related to each theme. The criteria specified were "generic" in nature because the criteria applied to clinicians in all six disciplines. These generic criteria were then reviewed by members of each discipline, who enhanced them to better reflect a particular discipline's practice and to distinguish among practice levels. With this refinement completed, the work of the professional development committee ended, and the focus moved to implementation. (Refer to Appendix B for levels of practice and behaviors for each discipline.)

The Implementation Process

As part of the implementation process, the Structure and Process Subcommittee identified the process and portfolio requirements for the four levels and the makeup and role of the review and appeals board process. The Education Subcommittee developed the plan to educate clinicians and leadership, and the Marketing Subcommittee addressed the issues of marketing and communication of the program.

The Implementation Committee used various approaches to inform and educate NPCS leaders and staff about the CRP. Early outreach efforts targeted clinical leaders. Gaining their support was considered crucial because those individuals would need to recognize staff at the Entry and Clinician levels as well as coach and endorse clinicians at the Advanced Clinician and Clinical Scholar levels. The senior vice president and chief nurse held a retreat with more than 100 clinical and administrative leaders, which was followed by additional group sessions and individual consultations. Educational sessions were held for the Review Board and Appeals Board to ensure there was a consistent understanding of the levels and criteria of the CRP.

In April 2002, the CRP was officially launched, and the Implementation Committee was replaced by a Steering Committee that was charged with overseeing CRP operations, monitoring the new program's effectiveness, and continuing its ongoing development. In the years since, the program has changed in response to feedback from clinicians and leadership. Nothing that occurred was unexpected given the culture change of implementing a program as large as the CRP, but at each challenge the NPCS leadership and clinicians chose to focus on improving and redesigning the program rather than reinventing it.

We have learned from our work in implementing a narrative culture that ensuring attention to the CRP must be ongoing. Today, the CRP plays an important role in the professional development of NPCS clinicians, and work is underway to expand the program to other disciplines, including Chaplaincy. What has been most significant has been the program's effect on the way clinicians and directors discuss clinical practice. The CRP has not only promoted a narrative culture and created more opportunities for examining practice but has also given directors and staff a language to discuss practice and clinical excellence—a language that is shared within and across all disciplines in NPCS.

In Their Own Words

The rest of this book includes the narratives of clinicians at MGH, but we believe these stories are much like stories that you might hear where you work. The authors of these narratives, who are probably similar to the clinicians you work with, will tell you what they did was nothing special—it was what anyone would do. We, like you, know that this is not true, but it is true that we often take for granted the exquisite compassionate care they deliver. We know the clinicians will deliver that care, and so we often stand back and watch rather than actively engage with the clinicians to understand what they are thinking as they care for this patient in that situation at that moment. It is in this questioning that the clinicians reflect and make their practice visible to themselves, their colleagues, and the organization.

Following each narrative is a brief commentary, which we provide to highlight key elements and skill in the narrative. The questions that follow—which we hope are similar to the questions you might have had while reading the narrative—are designed to be used to promote reflection and learning by the reader.

We know that one cannot write all one knows. We know the challenge in describing the exact moment when the patient is ready to learn, the feel of the ambu bag as one tries to oxygenate a patient in respiratory distress, or the feeling one gets when one knows "something is wrong." The only way we can understand the practice is by being curious and interested enough to ask questions and then be patient enough to listen to the answers.

Summary

The goal of this chapter is to show how one hospital's initial decision to incorporate narratives into its culture has continued to inform and strengthen its professional practice environment almost two decades later. The simplicity of the intervention, telling a story that has meaning in your practice, has allowed disciplines to focus on a shared goal—the desire for excellent patient care— and allowed leaders to understand and influence the practice environment in a new way.

Using the narrative as a foundation, MGH NPCS has created a recognition model that provides a pathway for professional development and the articulation of clinical expertise.

None of this work was easy, nor is the work complete, but it does continue. As MGH NPCS continues to create innovative models of care, we look beyond the metrics to the lived experience of what these changes mean. We listen to the narratives of patients and clinicians to identify themes and patterns, watching for signs of success or stress and making adjustments along the way.

References

Benner, P. (1984). *From novice to expert: Excellence and power in clinical nursing practice.* Menlo Park, CA: Addison-Wesley.

Benner, P., Hooper-Kyriakidis, P., & Stannard, D. (2011). *Clinical wisdom and interventions in acute and critical care: A thinking-in-action approach* (2nd ed.). Philadelphia, PA: W.B. Saunders.

Benner, P., Sutphen, M., Leonard, V., & Day, L. (2010). *Educating nurses: A call for radical transformation.* San Francisco, CA: Jossey-Boss.

Benner, P., Sutphen, M., Leonard-Kahn, V., & Day, L. (2008). Formation and everyday ethical comportment. *American Journal of Critical Care, 17*(5), 473–476.

Benner, P., Tanner, C., & Chesla, C. (1996). Expertise in nursing practice caring. *Clinical Judgment and Ethics.* New York City, NY: Springer Publishing.

Cathcart, E., & Greenspan, M. (2012). A new window on nurse manager development: Teaching for the practice. *The Journal of Nursing Administration, 42*(12), 557–561.

Cathcart, E., & Greenspan, M. (2013). The role of practical wisdom in nurse manager practice: Why experience matters. *The Journal of Nursing Administration, 21*(10), 964–970.

Dreyfus, H. L., & Dreyfus, S. E., with Athanasiou, T. (1986). *Mind over machine.* New York, NY: Free Press.

Paynton, S. (2009). The informal power of nurses for promoting patient care. *OJIN: The Online Journal of Issues in Nursing, 14*(1). Retrieved from http://www.nursingworld.org/MainMenuCategories/ANAMarketplace/ANAPeriodicals/OJIN/TableofContents/Vol142009/No1Jan09/ArticlePreviousTopic/InformalPowerofNurses.html

Riessman, C. K., & Quinney, L. (2005). Narrative in social work, a critical review. *Qualitative Social Work, 4*(4), 391–412.

Schultz, K., & Ravitch, S. M. (2013). Narratives of learning to teach: Taking on professional identities. *Journal of Teacher Education, 64*(1), 35–46.

Chapter 2

Theme of Practice: Clinician–Patient Relationship

*The interpersonal engagement or relational connection
between the clinician and the patient and/or family.*

The Importance of the Clinician–Patient Relationship

The theme of clinician–patient relationship was the first theme that was evident in the narratives that members of the Professional Development Committee reviewed. This was not surprising because central to the work of all clinicians in Patient Care Services is the care of patients and families. It is through the direct care of patients that clinicians gain a greater understanding of the following:

- Who the patient is

- Their unique needs and concerns

- Their lives beyond the walls of the institution

- The values and beliefs that give their lives meaning

This understanding allows the clinician to enter the patient's world and allows care to take place.

Narratives—Entry Level of Practice

At the Entry level of practice, the newly licensed clinician is learning how to establish a therapeutic relationship with patients and families. At this level clinicians are recognizing the differences among individuals in their response to illness and incorporating those differences in how they care and interact with the patient and family.

Narratives—Clinician Level of Practice

At the Clinician level of practice, the clinician is able to personalize the care of each patient and advocate for the patient and family. At this level the clinicians are able to incorporate individual and family needs into their interventions and plan of care.

Narratives—Advanced Clinician Level of Practice

At the Advanced Clinician level of practice, the clinicians have a deep understanding of patient/family dynamics and is able to incorporate complex factors into the plan of care. They advocate for the needs of patients and families and for the unit-based systems that support and influence care delivery.

Narratives—Clinical Scholar Level of Practice

At the Clinical Scholar level of practice, the Clinical Scholar advocates and empowers patients and families to maximize their participation in decision-making. The Clinical Scholar's influence moves beyond the unit/department and is felt organizationally.

Developing a therapeutic relationship is not innate; it is a skill that requires practice, experience, and reflection. For the newer clinician, building this skill begins by gaining confidence and comfort in working with patients and learning how to develop open, nonjudgmental behaviors with patients who have cultures and values different from the clinician's. The ability to understand and then incorporate those unique elements of the patient's life into his or her care, treatment, and planning is a key developmental milestone for the clinician. Continued experience and reflection allows the clinician to individualize his or her care and interactions based on the patient's needs.

The relationship with the patient allows the clinician to advocate for the patient with other members of the team within and beyond the walls of the institution. With newer clinicians, advocating for patients often mirrors the associated tasks and responsibilities required to structure the day. As the clinicians gain greater comfort and confidence in their skills and tasks, they are able to "see" the needs of the patient and act in a manner that influences their care, not just as individuals, but also for patients across the organization.

The narratives that follow describe the clinician–patient relationship across the six disciplines and across the four levels of expertise, as described in Chapter 1. The unbundling through reflective questions, which follows a brief commentary on the narrative, allows you to reflect on your own practice or that of a colleague.

Learning to Care for the Other Patient—The Family

David De La Hoz, RN   **Practice level: Entry**
Clinical Nurse, Medical Intensive Care

Since coming to work as a new graduate nurse, every single day has been full of new experiences. As nurses, we all know that when caring for our patients, the whole family needs to be included. Every patient has a different situation and family dynamic, and every family plays a significant role in our practice. Incorporating families into the plan of care can have a powerful impact on a patient's hospital course.

One Monday morning, my preceptor, Richard, and I received report from the night shift nurse on Mr. Adams. The first thing that stood out for me about Mr. Adams was that he had been diagnosed with a disease called *hereditary hemorrhagic telangiectasia* (HHT). I vaguely recalled this disease from my pathophysiology class in nursing school. Aside from what the name of the disease suggests (hemorrhaging as a result of hereditary disease), I did not remember anything else about it.

Richard shared that he had cared for patients with this disease in the past. He explained that HHT (which has autosomal-dominant inheritance) causes abnormally formed blood vessels. These abnormal blood vessels are usually found around the mouth, nose, and lips. And many patients with HHT also have arteriovenous malformations (AVMs) in the body's internal organs, such as in the GI tract, liver, lungs, brain, and/or the spine.

Mr. Adams's wife brought him to the hospital after he experienced yet another bleed. He suffered a massive upper-GI bleed and was vomiting blood. His EGD (endoscopic exam) revealed an entire liter of blood in his stomach. From the moment I met Mrs. Adams, I could tell that she was extremely anxious—fearful that her husband would re-bleed and that it would go undetected. I reassured her we were monitoring his vital signs very closely, and we would know immediately if his status changed. Unfortunately, it didn't do much to alleviate her concerns.

Mrs. Adams was adamant that she could tell when her husband was going to have a bleed because she knew certain "warning signs." I saw this as a window of opportunity to alleviate her anxiety. I asked her to tell me about his warning signs. She explained that there were subtle cues that preceded each bleed and she was acutely attuned to recognizing them. After talking about the warning signs for several minutes, she appeared to relax just a little.

Although her overall anxiety abated, Mrs. Adams still panicked whenever Mr. Adams did anything out of the ordinary, such as cough or sigh. I tried to think of something I could do to help her relax.

Again, I offered her reassurance and explained our monitoring system. Even though I was repeating the same information I had told her earlier, this time it seemed to bring her relief. She said, "Thank you for explaining that to me."

I realized that her elevated level of anxiety had prevented her from hearing or comprehending what I said the first time. I made a mental note that Mrs. Adams would require ongoing reassurance and explanations.

Soon, Richard returned and asked Mrs. Adams a question that hadn't even crossed my mind. He asked how long it had been since she'd gone home to rest or have a meal. Mrs. Adams said that she hadn't slept since the night before she brought Mr. Adams to the emergency department. We realized that Mrs. Adams hadn't left her husband's side except for bathroom breaks since he arrived.

Richard took that as the opportunity to help Mrs. Adams understand why it was important for her to take care of herself, as well. Even though her husband was very sick and in the ICU, she needed to make sure she got enough rest and nourishment, too. His words fell onto receptive ears because Mrs. Adams immediately went down to the cafeteria and had a good lunch. When she returned about 45 minutes later, she looked almost like a different person.

Mrs. Adams was more relaxed that afternoon, but still somewhat anxious. I recalled that in nursing school they engrained in us the importance of involving the patient's family in the care of the patient. I tried to think of ways Mrs. Adams could participate in caring for her husband. I started with the most basic activity—washing and combing his hair. Mrs. Adams was thrilled to have something contributory to do. She had felt helpless sitting in the background watching everyone else care for Mr. Adams. She said she was the one who provided all his care at home.

Throughout the day Mrs. Adams became progressively more relaxed, and by the end of our shift, she thanked us for helping her husband so much. I like to think it was the small things, like listening to her, reassuring her, showing empathy, and involving her in her husband's care that had such a positive impact on Mrs. Adams.

Commentary

Patients and families place tremendous trust in their caregivers. That trust is not conferred simply by being in a role or from the name of an institution. Trust comes from relationships. Patients and families are hypervigilant to the care, commitment, and the skill of their care team as clinicians and support staff take the time to "know" them.

As a new graduate nurse, David's focus was correctly attuned to the complexities inherent in caring for a patient as ill as Mr. Adams. But he also recognized the anxiety his wife was experiencing and sought to decrease her anxiety and fear by recognizing her important role not only as Mr. Adams's wife, but also as caregiver.

Richard's role as preceptor is highlighted in not only teaching David the clinical skills needed in learning the practice but also in the further development of caring practices that support the healing of all members of the family.

Reflective Questions

- David actively involved Mrs. Adams in the direct care of her husband. How do you know to offer this as an option to family members? What if those family members do not react well to your offer?

- As a new registered nurse in the ICU, David had to search his memory for what Mr. A's diagnosis was and how it would inform his care. What resources do you use to help learn about these complex diagnoses and interventions you are seeing for the first time?

- Patients and families are often anxious being in the hospital. How do you address any questions or concerns they might have being cared for by a new registered nurse?

Opening the Door—#1

Susan Ross, LICSW   **Practice level: Clinician**
Clinical Social Worker, Cardiac Surgical Intensive Care and Step-Down

Critically ill patients in the Cardiac Surgical ICU are in a vulnerable place, facing issues beyond their experience. I feel privileged to have had the opportunity to support one such patient as she faced the end of her life. Michelle was brought emergently to MGH after an acute myocardial infarction, which led to a long and complicated stay in the Cardiac Surgical ICU. Michelle was placed on extra-corporeal membrane oxygenation (ECMO) in the operating room and remained critically ill throughout her hospitalization.

During my initial visits with Michelle, she would lie in bed with the covers up to her chin and stare at the ceiling. She would briefly acknowledge my presence and express feeling thankful that she had survived. With further exploration, Michelle shared that she didn't feel ready to "face this reality." I validated those feelings and tried to focus on building rapport and trust. To develop our therapeutic alliance, I met with Michelle on a regular basis; she felt comfortable enough with me to vent her feelings and fears.

When I asked how she had coped with challenges in the past, she just looked at me and said, "I pushed it all away." Then she shook her head and began to sob. I sat with her as she cried and created a space where she could begin to explore her feelings and allow herself to be vulnerable. I wanted her to know that I would remain present, supportive, and open as she went through this challenging time.

As our rapport grew stronger, my work with Michelle began to focus on developing her ability to cope with her serious and progressive health issues. She had a history of detaching and internalizing her feelings, but due to the acuity of this situation she felt forced to face the reality of her physical illness. She began to share details of her social history, opening up to me about her 19-year-old daughter and her daughter's struggle with a severe learning disability; her boyfriend, who was dependent on her financially and emotionally; and the distant relationships she had with her brother and sister.

During the time I spent with Michelle, many of her interpersonal struggles and feelings of guilt at not being able to continue in these relationships began to emerge. Michelle's lack of control became a common theme. Her acute illness and complex family dynamics became an emotionally draining and time-consuming situation both for Michelle and for staff involved in her care.

I helped Michelle articulate her needs and wishes. Over time, with Michelle's input, the interdisciplinary team and I found creative ways to increase her sense of control. We created a schedule that her nurses updated regularly with her goals for the day. This helped Michelle track her progress and empowered her to be part of her care planning.

Michelle experienced great anxiety, which became more debilitating over time, ultimately impacting her ability to sleep and tolerate daily interventions. At times, her anxiety escalated to where she described tightness in her chest and difficulty breathing. When it passed, I'd ask Michelle how I could support her during those times, to which she replied, "Just being present." I consulted with the psychiatric clinical nurse specialist about the impact of Michelle's anxiety on her care, and she began to meet with Michelle to teach her how to practice relaxation techniques.

As Michelle continued to physically deteriorate, opportunities arose for us to discuss her fears and struggles related to her mortality. The Cardiac Surgery and Palliative Care teams shared with Michelle that her prognosis was increasingly poor, which led to discussions about goals of care. After these conversations, Michelle would openly express her fears about dying. To help her manage her anxiety, I asked her to let me know if she began to feel overwhelmed. This helped inform how to safely increase her distress tolerance and gave her a sense of control over the direction of our time together.

She shared her concerns about whether her daughter and boyfriend would be able to manage if she didn't survive or was unable to be active in their lives. Michelle wanted to work on her relationships with her brother and sister. With her guidance, we engaged in conversations with her siblings where she expressed her hopes that they would be more involved with her daughter and boyfriend. She shared with them her fears about the future. These discussions were difficult for Michelle, but therapeutic in being able to join together as a family to prepare and address these concerns.

Michelle struggled with the idea of leaving her daughter.

The question for me became, "What does it mean to Michelle to say good-bye?" Her focus was on sorting out her daughter's and boyfriend's social and financial needs. She wanted to know they'd be taken care of if she didn't survive. Michelle spoke with her brother and sister about coordinating services, such as disability income and housing for her daughter, which she had intended to do herself. Her siblings assured her that these matters would be taken care of, and I provided them with information about these resources. Michelle's sister invited her daughter to move in with her until she could find an apartment, and Michelle's boyfriend moved in with a close friend who could share expenses.

Michelle passed away after suffering a stroke almost two months after being admitted. My hope is that Michelle felt her voice was heard at the end of her life. She was able to explore the prospect of leaving her child and seize the opportunity to make arrangements for her daughter's ongoing safety and well-being. My work with Michelle helped me realize the power of being present and open to a person's fears and anxieties at the end of life. As a new social worker, working with Michelle helped me focus on the therapeutic alliance and showed me how a strong foundation can present opportunities for self-exploration, both for the patient and the social worker. The most rewarding aspect of my job is being able to have an impact on patients' lives during their most vulnerable and challenging times.

Commentary

Susan met Michelle at a point at which she could no longer hide from the reality of her illness and what her death would mean to those she loved. Through Susan's presence, skill, and compassion, she actively assisted Michelle with managing her anxiety and sorting out family issues, including giving her control of when the conversation needed to end if it provoked too much anxiety. The level of trust that Susan was able to develop empowered Michelle to gain a level of peace and calm as she moved to acceptance of her death.

Reflective Questions

- Michelle brings up many regrets and fears as she negotiates the end of her life. How would you help Michelle face those regrets and fears?

- Susan helped Michelle take control and advocate for herself. Why is that important?

- To get patients to open up to you, it's critical to develop a relationship of trust. What's the first thing you need to do to begin developing a trust relationship? What do you need to do to sustain that relationship?

People Will Surprise You

Tessa Rowin, PT
Physical Therapist

Practice level: Clinician

In my clinical practice, I have had the privilege of meeting patients from all walks of life; from a variety of cultures, races, and ethnicities; and from a vast spectrum of socioeconomic backgrounds. Each patient comes to the hospital, and specifically to physical therapy, with a variety of experiences and beliefs that impact the plan of care but do not necessarily predict the outcome or final prognosis of Physical Therapy (PT) intervention. A few months ago, I had the pleasure of meeting Mr. Petersen, who helped me understand this factor and how to incorporate this understanding into my clinical decision-making.

Mr. Petersen is a 56-year-old gentleman who was referred to physical therapy for chronic back and leg pain. He has an extensive past medical history, for which he has been treated at numerous facilities. He also had a long list of missed appointments. The assessment from his referring physician was as follows: "56-year-old male with multiple vague symptoms who is convinced he has a lot of medical conditions that have not been verified. Back/leg pain: symptoms likely related to sciatica." From the initial chart review, my biased impression was that physical therapy was unlikely to make a difference in this patient's symptoms, but a complete evaluation was clearly necessary.

At the initial evaluation with Mr. Petersen, I took my usual subjective history, attempting not only to gain information regarding Mr. Petersen's symptoms but also to get to know him as a person. Mr. Petersen had been unemployed for some time and lived in a group home, related to his being homeless. Mr. Petersen was not a great historian and had difficulty being specific about activities that intensified or improved his chronic symptoms of back and leg pain. What he described did not fit a musculoskeletal pattern, and he reported no success with treatment in the past. He also was quite vocal about his difficulty with other providers and felt that he really wasn't receiving care that was improving any of his symptoms. I have seen a handful of patients with similar stories for whom PT prognosis had been guarded and past experiences had hindered PT participation. My pattern recognition set in, and my gut was telling me that this relationship and physical therapy intervention was not going to lead to significant functional gains.

I proceeded to perform a full examination of Mr. Petersen —watching him mobilize and testing impairments that could potentially be aggravating his symptoms. By the end of the session, I had determined that he likely had some changes to his spine that could be contributing to the limitations I was observing. I instructed him in two basic exercises to improve mobility and posture. Despite my initial bias regarding PT prognosis, I spent a good amount of time explaining the role of physical therapy and what my expectations were for both myself and for him to optimize his functional outcome and reach his goals. At the end of the session, I thought to myself, "I wonder if Mr. Petersen will ever return."

Sure enough, Mr. Petersen did not show up for his next two appointments. A week later I received two voicemails from Mr. Petersen stating that he had conflicts and would not be able to make his next appointment. He reported that he had no phone, but he knew that he had one scheduled visit left and that he would be there. Mr. Petersen did not come to that appointment. I assumed he was lost to follow-up because I did not have any way to contact him.

One month later, Mr. Petersen was back on my schedule, and I was surprised when he did show up. I was preparing to have a conversation with him to tell him that inconsistency of follow-up with PT would not lead to the outcome he wanted, but when Mr. Petersen came back to the treatment area, he explained to me that there were extenuating circumstances that had caused him to miss his appointments. Despite missing those appointments, Mr. Petersen told me that he had been doing his exercises all along, and they were actually helping him manage his pain. This took me by surprise, and I was quite happy to hear that he had taken to heart our initial discussion. We went through a progression of exercises, and when he returned the next week he reported resolution of his distal symptoms and felt that he was making gradual improvements.

Unfortunately, I did not have the opportunity to follow up again with Mr. Petersen, as he missed his last visit and did not reschedule. However, I can imagine that given his motivation and improvements with the initial set of exercises, he would continue working to improve his posture and flexibility to ultimately improve his functional mobility.

This case truly made me appreciate the time I spend educating patients about their conditions and explaining why I believe physical therapy treatment is a good decision at the given time. I realized that my initial doubts and bias against this patient because of his background and history with other healthcare providers could have clouded my initial judgment about his potential progress with PT. However, I knew that my interpersonal skills had clearly trumped my inner thoughts when Mr. Petersen returned after 6 weeks and showed me that he was faithful with those initial two exercises.

This demonstrates the value of the patient–clinician relationship and the ability to advocate for what is in the best interest of the patient despite prior encounters with healthcare professionals. Although I always attempt to be open-minded, pattern recognition for past successes or failures has a role in clinical decision-making regarding expectations of outcome. My appreciation of avoiding initial judgment has been heightened, and I hope to always remember with my future patients to give the benefit of the doubt.

Commentary

What's the old adage? You can't judge a book by its cover? Never is it truer than when talking about patient care. It can be difficult for clinicians to admit that preconceived assumptions affect their judgment, but we've all done it. Tessa's expertise and bravery in sharing this narrative allows each of us to ask when our preconceived assumptions caused us to be blind to the possibility of another story. This narrative reminds us to use our powers of observation, clinical decision-making, and the gift of curiosity, which enables us to ask more questions, wonder, and see possibilities.

Reflective Questions

- Tessa was very aware that reading Mr. Petersen's record and listening to him describe past failures with PT made her believe that Mr. Petersen would not adhere to his scheduled visits or treatment plan. How do you overcome such judgments about patients?

- Mr. Petersen told Tessa that other providers had not helped him. If a patient defines success as cure, and that is not possible, how do you work with the patient to redefine success?

- Have you ever been in a situation where you felt your treatment plan would not actually help the patient? What do you do in such situations?

The Middle Way

Nicole Martinez, RN
Clinical Nurse, Psychiatry

Practice level: Advanced Clinician

On the inpatient Psychiatric Unit, we are no strangers to psychogenic pain. Sometimes a patient's pain has a medical origin; sometimes it's idiopathic. Javier's was a bit of both. He had experienced severe, recurrent, abdominal pain over the last year that hadn't responded well to medical interventions. His pain seemed disproportionate to the cause.

As a nurse, I'm not immune to the frustrations that accompany incurable illness. I've learned to adapt to accommodate the needs of my patients. The question may become, "How am I going to help my patient live with pain?" versus, "How am I going to relieve the pain?" The answer is not always simple and must be tailored to the needs of each patient. In Javier's case, he needed to be understood as a whole person, not just as someone with a severe, unmanageable reaction to pain.

I first met Javier 4 years ago when he became suicidal after receiving a new HIV diagnosis. I remembered being surprised at how quickly he improved; he was discharged within 2 days.

Javier was readmitted last year for treatment of suicidal ideation related to pain. His condition had deteriorated. He previously had several admissions to local emergency departments for severe abdominal pain. He had undergone numerous medical and surgical treatments, including a cholecystectomy, fluid collections in the gall bladder, H. pylori, candidal esophagitis, bi-ductal sphincterotomy, and placement of a stent. His current diagnosis was CMV esophagitis with sphincter dysfunction. Javier hoped that stent-removal surgery would resolve his pain.

As he waited for surgery, Javier experienced severe bouts of pain. I'd find him crying, huddled in a fetal position in the bathroom. He wouldn't ask for medication, because he knew it wouldn't help. Narcotics would only make him more constipated and lead to more pain. He'd been seen by the Pain Service team several times. Instead of asking for help, he seemed to want to hide.

I advised Javier to try guided imagery. I asked him to imagine a safe place (he chose a mountain) where he could feel more relaxed. He enjoyed the exercise and thought he could revisit it on his own. We spoke about mindfulness meditation and the effect it has on dealing with pain. I advised him to meditate for a few minutes every day and notice what affect it had on his pain.

His occupational therapist added sensory-based coping strategies to counteract his pain. We encouraged him to use squeeze balls and bite towels to draw the pain away from him. He took warm showers when he felt pain starting. These techniques were especially helpful during acute bouts of pain. I recommended Reiki and Therapeutic Touch to balance the energy in his body and help it heal. These techniques have been effective in treating pain, especially when administered by an experienced practitioner.

I encouraged Javier to attend group sessions on the unit to learn more coping techniques and share his struggle with others. He had very few social contacts outside his family. Typically, when patients make social contacts, they're more apt to eat in the day room and attend group activities.

Javier continued to experience pain. It became worse when he ate certain foods and, as a Type II diabetic, when he was hypo- or hyperglycemic. He didn't adhere to a good diabetic diet outside the hospital; many of his meals were at the kitchen of the hotel where he worked, and mostly after 3:00 p.m., when his shift started. Javier loved food, and even though he was in pain, he'd eat anything fried or greasy that was put in front of him. Knowing this, I consulted our nutritionist. We reviewed Javier's eating habits and medical condition, and she encouraged him to eat six small meals a day and avoid fried, fatty, and greasy foods. We encouraged him to try to adhere to a bowel regimen of one bowel movement a day. I worked with him to improve compliance; we recorded his input, output, finger sticks, and how he felt after meals. I placed a lot of emphasis on education, and we worked on a diet that would fit his lifestyle. Javier responded well to this approach and was surprised at how much it impacted his pain level. But despite this, his main focus continued to be surgery.

Though Javier had many challenges, I wanted him to appreciate his strengths. Chronic pain can be all consuming, and Javier was becoming blind to the good things in his life. I encouraged him to examine his life, focusing on the positive.

He was devoted to his family. He had a teenage son and three adult children. He was proud that his grown sons would hug and kiss him in public. He enjoyed good relationships with his sisters, who lived nearby. He spoke flawless English (though English wasn't his native language). He had a job he enjoyed. Javier agreed that these were all reasons to keep living and keep fighting.

I met frequently with Javier to talk about his depression. I knew from his previous admission that he'd contracted HIV during a period of promiscuity after his wife left him. He spoke very little about his ex-wife or how the end of their relationship affected him. He believed his depression stemmed from witnessing his father's death 20 years before. His father had been terminally ill and died in his arms. He never got over it and hasn't been able to be truly happy since. He thought of it as a form of post-traumatic stress, with nightmares and a sense of being disconnected from others. His psychiatric medications were adjusted to target pain pathways and post-traumatic stress.

Because he was self-reflective and had good reasoning skills, his psychologist and I thought he would be a perfect candidate for talk therapy. I encouraged him to reflect on his experiences during his hospitalization and share them with me and other staff members.

The night before Javier was scheduled to go home, I received a call from Gastroenterology. He was booked for surgery the following day. He was going to have the surgery he so desperately wanted. I asked the doctor if he thought the surgery would decrease his pain, and he said no.

One thing I've learned as a psychiatric nurse is not to take away a patient's hope, but I didn't want to give Javier false promises, so I decided to try what Buddhists call "the middle way." I gave him a pep talk. I told Javier he was going to be discharged soon, and I probably wouldn't see him again after this shift. I told him his life would continue to be a struggle at times, but to be proud of the work he'd done. I told him he was going to have surgery in the morning, and his eyes lit up as if he'd just won the lottery.

He asked me if I thought the surgery would "work," and I carefully replied, "If you believe it will, then it just might." He thanked me for my care and said he'd include my comment in his journal. "I'll think about that," he said.

As a psychiatric nurse, I see patients for a short time only. For me, it's about planting a seed of knowledge that can further their personal development. It's not about "fixing" someone, but providing them with tools they can use to cope with the chronicity of their illness. I imagine Javier may still have pain. But I hope he'll see the value in seeking help from healthcare providers and using some of what he learned as he progresses through the continuum of his life.

Commentary

We frequently use terms such as "success" and "failure," but often, in reality, life falls somewhere in between. Empowered by understanding and compassion, Nicole gently guided Javier to live his life as fully as he was able. She cared for him, advocated for him, and educated him. She gave him the tools to discover aspects of his care that he could control. Recognizing the limits and risks of medication, she was open to holistic interventions that could have eased Javier's pain and assisted him in managing stress after he left the hospital. The narrative reflects Nicole's comfort in situations that have no clear-cut answer. She gave Javier so much; perhaps more than anything, she gave him hope.

Reflective Questions

- In collaboration with the occupational therapist, Nicole utilized multiple sensory modification techniques to help Javier manage his pain. Have such techniques been effective for your patients? Are there techniques that work better for some patients than others?

- What do you know about the "middle way," which is a path of moderation? How might you use this idea to help patients?

- Nicole describes the need for patients to have hope. How do you help your patients find hope in situations where they may not be able to even consider the possibility of hope?

Bridging Cultures, Taking Risks

Janet Actis, RN
Clinical Nurse, Pediatrics

Practice level: Advanced Clinician

Being a pediatric nurse is so rewarding, especially when you witness the resiliency of children. Many children recover against great odds, but unfortunately, some lose their battles. No one can teach a nurse what to do in those situations. It's an innate quality a nurse has and discovers as she or he comforts families and assists in giving a child a peaceful and dignified passing. Caring for Mingzhu and his family helped me find this quality in myself and enhance my practice as a pediatric nurse.

My experience with Mingzhu and his family taught me a great deal about Chinese culture, including their views on life and death and how decisions are made within the family. The Chinese culture looks to its elders for direction. It views death as a positive thing for elders and a negative thing for children. I happened to be precepting a new graduate nurse at the time, Elise, and it was her first end-of-life experience as a nurse.

Mingzhu was transferred to our general pediatric unit from the hematology-oncology clinic. I was the resource nurse that day. Mingzhu's nurse in the clinic informed me that he was a 6-year-old boy with an abdominal rhabdomyosarcoma (solid tumor) who'd been treated with chemotherapy, radiation, and surgery in China but hadn't responded, so he was brought to Boston as a last hope. Because Mingzhu did not speak any English, Mingzhu's parents and paternal grandparents accompanied him on the trip. Mingzhu's pain was increasing, and to add to an already stressful situation, Mingzhu's mom was 8 months pregnant.

At first, I helped other nurses with creative ways to care for Mingzhu and his family. The entire team truly came together. I helped arrange a sonogram at his bedside so he could see his baby sister, as this was his last request, to live long enough to see his new sister. Soon it was decided that Mingzhu would be brought to the home of a friend in the area to receive hospice care.

I was his nurse the day before he was to be discharged. As Mingzhu's mom and I rode down in the elevator to get his medications from the pharmacy, she told me (in her limited English) about the comic books Mingzhu loved. She was so grateful for our efforts to transfer him out of the hospital. As the day progressed, Mingzhu's pain returned and, with the aid of an interpreter, the oncologist again explained to Mingzhu's parents that we could make him comfortable, but we couldn't make him better.

For whatever reason, this time they really understood what it meant. I had my arms around Mingzhu's mom as she sobbed. Mingzhu's dad, who hadn't touched Mingzhu much before, held his son like it was the last time he ever would. Mingzhu's mom asked to speak to the oncologist, the interpreter, and me outside.

She said, "I cannot ask this in front of my husband, but how much time do we have?" I knew then that Mingzhu's mom understood, and she had more strength than I imagined—8 months pregnant and caring for her whole family at this difficult time. Unfortunately, Mingzhu did not have much time at all.

Mingzhu's family avoided questions about their wishes for final arrangements. Gradually I came to understand that in the Chinese culture, a child's death is a "black death," unlike an elder's death, which is considered a "white death" because the person had a chance to live a full life and gain wisdom. Not only was I concerned about how Mingzhu's family was coping with his impending death, I was worried about how my preceptee, Elise, was doing. I encouraged her to share her feelings with me or any other veteran nurses.

When Mingzhu's last day came, for whatever reason, I knew it was the day. The family informed us that they would need new clothes for Mingzhu for all seasons. As part of their cultural tradition, we would need to dress him to prepare him for the afterlife.

Mingzhu passed away comfortably, surrounded by his family. We helped them wash and dress him in his new clothes so his spirit would be ready for the afterlife. We let the family grieve and pray together.

Arrangements were made per Chinese tradition to allow Mingzhu to stay on the unit an extra day to give the family time to grieve. If he were taken away sooner, they would be robbed of the opportunity to grieve their loss and begin to heal. According to custom, after this grieving period, no one speaks of the child or his death. We made arrangements with the funeral home (whose director spoke Mandarin) for Mingzhu to be picked up the next day. Our Mandarin interpreters helped staff understand the cultural aspects of this practice, which helped me provide better care for Mingzhu and his family.

I knew Mingzhu's mom was due to deliver any time. I came in the next morning (a Sunday) still grieving Mingzhu's death, but I had to help the family navigate through this unknown time. When the time came for him to be taken to the funeral home, they said one last good-bye at the end of the hallway, and I slowly helped the family leave the unit for the first time without their son. I hoped they would be able to embrace the joy of their new daughter, who would be born soon. Sooner, in fact, than any of us thought.

A few hours later, I turned to see Mingzhu's mom and dad were there, with the aid of a friend, and that Mingzhu's mom was having break-through bleeding. I instructed them to go straight to Labor and Delivery, as we had practiced before Mingzhu died, and she was quickly admitted. When I went up to check on them later, as I came out of the elevator, I saw Mingzhu's grandparents looking lost and confused. When they saw me, the stress disappeared—I was a familiar face in a foreign setting. I helped them all reunite, and we learned the next morning that Mingzhu's mom would be induced after she got some rest.

As individuals, we have our own beliefs. But as nurses, we're taught to be open to hearing about our patients' and families' beliefs. That can be difficult in emotionally charged situations, and especially when people of different cultures come together. One thing that helped was collaborating with the pediatric palliative care team who came and spoke to the staff about Mingzhu's impending death, our feelings, and how the family's culture impacted our care. This helped me to be more sensitive to each member of Mingzhu's family and to understand the family dynamics from a cultural perspective.

When I reflect on Mingzhu's death, his transfer to the funeral home, helping Mingzhu's parents to Labor and Delivery, and helping his grandparents find them, I realize the significance of the help I was able to provide. But, truthfully, Mingzhu and his family gave me so much more than I gave them. It was only after I got home Sunday night that I realized how special and unique this situation was. I'd never heard of a child staying on a unit 24 hours after dying. It would be the last thing I would want as a mother. But as nurses we can put our own feelings aside. And as difficult as that may have been, I now understand how, culturally, it was the right thing to do for Mingzhu and his family. I now understand the impact nurses can have by going the extra mile, supporting one another, and providing care that's culturally competent and sensitive. I'm proud that I found the ability in myself to help ease the loss of a child and support this family with a culturally dignified death.

Commentary

Janet's skill and compassion are evident in every paragraph of this narrative. She was constantly alert to Mingzhu's family's needs as well as those of her preceptee. She anticipated, intervened, and altered the environment to ensure that this devastating loss was handled with dignity and in a way that respected the family's long-held customs and beliefs—even when those beliefs didn't coincide with her own. This was a valuable life and nursing lesson, one I'm sure Janet will carry with her for the rest of her career.

Reflective Questions

- In caring for patients, you often have to be respectful of a culture very different from what you know. How do you remain open and nonjudgmental? How do you ensure your colleagues are able to care for such patients and family members in the same manner?

- In Mingzhu's room there was the sadness of his pending death and the joy of the birth of his sister. What is it like to deal with such different emotions at the same time? What has helped you and your colleagues?

- The sensitivity and understanding to keep Mingzhu's body on the unit gave his family such peace. How do you create a culture where only one question is asked: Is this for the benefit of the patient and family?

The Do-Over

Melissa Mattola-Kiatos, RN
Clinical Nurse, Operating Room

Practice level: Advanced Clinician

I encountered a patient, Gina, who was to undergo a breast biopsy with needle localization; I was her circulating nurse in the operating room. A *circulating nurse* is a registered nurse who makes preparations for an operation and continually monitors the patient and staff during its course, works in the operating room outside the sterile field in which the operation takes place, records the progress of the operation, accounts for the instruments, and handles specimens. In reviewing Gina's record, I noted that she suffered from anxiety, which she occasionally managed with medication. I recognized that undergoing a biopsy could trigger anxiety in Gina.

I introduced myself to Gina and, after verifying her identity, immediately I started to have a conversation with her about nothing and everything. I noted that when she spoke about her children the nervous movements she made, such as hand-wringing and tapping her feet, lessened. I slowly steered the conversation back to the procedure that she was to undergo. As I was talking to Gina about her past surgical history, she told me that 5 weeks earlier she had had a surgical procedure and experienced a great deal of pain and anxiety afterward. I reviewed with her that, based on the attending surgeon's history and physical, the calcifications that we were removing from her breast today were fairly superficial, and the pain should not be as profound as when she had her previous surgery, which visibly calmed her.

I described what she would see and hear when she entered the operating room, careful to observe her response to the information I was giving her. I did not want to overwhelm her or make her more anxious, but because I had observed that information about what she could expect in postoperative pain calmed her, I continued my explanation. Gina took great comfort in hearing the steps of the procedure and knowing that she would be comfortably asleep before we started anything invasive; I assured her that we would take all of the steps necessary to make sure that she was comfortable and safe throughout the procedure. I also explained to her that the certified nurse anesthetist (CRNA) that was working with her would speak with her shortly, and I would be sure to convey to the CRNA the patient's concerns about pain management following surgery.

Gina and I spent some additional time together to discuss the overall procedure, and I answered any additional questions that she had. The CRNA arrived to speak with Gina, and after I introduced them to each other, I stepped away from the patient while the CRNA interviewed Gina to make sure that we had all of the necessary equipment in the operating room. I made a point to talk to Gina and tell her why I was going into the operating room, and that I would be back to see her before she entered the operating room to make sure that she didn't have any additional questions.

Following the CRNA's interview, I returned to Gina to make sure she didn't have any additional questions or need anything further, which she didn't. When all of the surgical team was present, we conducted our preoperative huddle prior to the procedure. During this huddle I expressed the patient's concerns regarding her anxiety and her pain management following the procedure. We discussed at length her concerns about not being able to control her pain and the additional anxiety that this concern was for her preoperatively. All members of the surgical team were then on the same page concerning Gina and her anxiety concerning the procedure and postoperative pain management.

When we brought Gina into the operating room, she was shaking slightly due to her nervousness. I stayed by her side and held her hand, which she gripped very tightly, and I explained to her everything that was going on around her in simple terms. Gina seemed to respond well to me speaking with her as somewhat of a distraction technique while she was being induced by anesthesia. She closed her eyes and took deep, even breaths to help relieve anxiety, and the grip that she held so tightly on my hand loosened. Throughout all of her induction, I held her hand and continued to provide reassurance to her. She then was sedated and was sleeping comfortably; her tight grip on my hand relaxed. Her procedure was being done as "monitored anesthesia care" (MAC), so she was not intubated.

Gina tolerated her procedure very well and began to awaken at the end of the procedure. I was immediately by her side and again providing some reassurance that she was safe and still in the operating room. She immediately became very awake and alert and kept saying to me, "Am I okay? I feel like I am going to jump out of my skin." Gina repeated these same words several times. I took hold of her hand and continued to reassure her that she was okay and that she was still in the operating room. The CRNA had also begun to intervene and had given Gina "something to relax her."

We helped Gina move to her stretcher for transport to the recovery room. She was sitting up in the stretcher and still kept repeating that she felt very anxious. I confirmed with Gina that she was feeling anxious and that she was not experiencing pain. About the same time that the procedure was ending, another nurse came into the operating room to offer me lunch. Under normal operating procedure in the operating room, the circulating nurse does not accompany the patient to the recovery room. However, I felt that, given the comfort that Gina seemed to take from my presence, my accompanying her to the Post Anesthesia Care Unit (PACU) would help to ease some of her anxiety. I also felt that I could act as a resource during transport that was solely dedicated to reassuring Gina and providing her with emotional support.

I accompanied the patient, resident, and CRNA to the recovery room. The entire time I was with Gina, I held her hand and continued to reassure her. We wheeled into the recovery bay in the PACU, and I introduced Gina to the nurse that was going to be her recovery room nurse. I had a conversation with the PACU nurse that included Gina and that detailed that she was feeling anxious following her procedure, but that she was practicing deep breathing and that she was starting to feel a little better. We also as a team discussed Gina's concerns about her pain management and her ongoing anxieties. Gina was an active participant in this interaction with the PACU nurse. By including Gina in the hand-off report with the PACU nurse, it helped to give her a sense of control of her situation and helped to ease some of her anxiety. After spending an additional 5 minutes or so with Gina, I felt that she was substantially more relaxed, and I felt very comfortable leaving her in the PACU. Gina thanked me for everything that I had done and told me that she wouldn't forget how much I helped her.

I followed up with Gina's attending surgeon about a week later to check in and see how she was doing. The timing of my inquiry could not have been more perfect. As it turned out, Gina was returning to the operating room that very day to have additional tissue excised. We discussed Gina's anxiety, and the surgeon confirmed she had prescribed some anti-anxiety medication that Gina could take the night before and the morning of surgery to assist her in controlling her anxiety.

I was in between cases and had the opportunity to visit the Center for Peri-Operative Care Unit (CPC) pre-op area prior to Gina's case to see if she was there. She was comfortably sitting in a stretcher and had a member of her family with her. Before I could even say hello to her, she recognized me, called my name, and introduced me to her aunt. Gina told me how grateful she was for everything that I had previously done for her; she also told me how her previous experience had helped to shape her current experience and that she was able to take something "to relax her" ahead of time. I wished Gina the best, and I was grateful that I had an opportunity to close the circle and follow up on her. Gina reminds me of why even small things and taking the time to listen can make a big impact on patients' experiences and expectations.

Commentary

If it were not for Melissa's recognition and interventions, Gina's underlying anxiety and past experience with postoperative pain could have set her up for a very challenging experience as she underwent her breast biopsy. Melissa began her interventions by taking time to know Gina as a person and then slowly and with attention and care introduced Gina to the OR team and environment. Making time for this is challenging in environments where time is of the essence, but Melissa made it happen. She was mindful of handoffs and consistently shared with all members of the team who Gina was and what she needed from all of them.

Reflective Questions

- Melissa was purposeful in how she gave Gina information and observed her reaction to it. How do you balance what you need to communicate to patients and how they are processing and reacting to it?

- Gina did not consistently rely on medication to help her manage her anxiety. How do you know when a patient needs medication versus using relaxation techniques?

- Is there a correlation between how patients "go to sleep" and how they wake up from anesthesia?

Empowerment

Shauna Harris, RN   **Practice level: Advanced Clinician**
Clinical Nurse, Obstetrics

In this narrative, I have the opportunity to reflect on an occasion when I became a clinical "Sherpa," guiding a patient and her family through obstacles complicated by differences in culture and beliefs. This story highlights the lasting impact nurses can have on patients despite the rapid turnover on the Newborn Family Unit.

Mrs. Sabate was a 36-year-old woman from Sudan and a devout Muslim. My initial meeting with her occurred when she delivered her third child about 2 years ago. During report from the nurse going off duty, I learned that Mrs. Sabate had a history of diabetes and obesity, which had the potential of complicating her delivery. Mrs. Sabate did not adhere to her diabetic regimen and treatment plan, even missing some of her prenatal appointments that were important to the ongoing monitoring of her health and her unborn child. During one ultrasound appointment, the baby's heart rate showed signs of distress. The recommendation was for Mrs. Sabate to have a C-section a few weeks before her due date.

Mrs. Sabate and her husband raised objections to a C-section based on their beliefs as Muslims. They both insisted it should be left to God to determine the time of delivery. Mr. Sabate was more vocal and somewhat aggressive when dealing with his wife's caregivers. Based on her missing appointments, her husband's aggressive behavior, the alarming decrease in the baby's heart rate and signs of distress, and the couple's unwillingness to have the C-section in the face of this potentially dire situation, the social worker was consulted. Following her evaluation, consultation with the entire team, and careful consideration, the social worker contacted the Department of Children and Families (DCF) due to concerns that the family's other young children were being neglected. The couple eventually agreed to the C-section, which was done without complication. However, despite the successful delivery, Mr. Sabate was furious about the social worker and the fact that DCF had been contacted, especially now that his wife had delivered a healthy child.

While listening to this report and hearing how nurses viewed the case, I decided it was key to remain unbiased. My plan was to express empathy, aware that cultural and religious beliefs could have accounted for the couple's approach to the situation. It was possible the husband's anger could have stemmed from anxiety about the birth and fear of the unknown.

I entered the room with a smile and greeted Mr. and Mrs. Sabate respectfully. Mrs. Sabate's English was limited, and even though Mr. Sabate spoke well enough and could translate, I opted to use a medical interpreter to communicate. This ensured that I heard from Mrs. Sabate directly about her needs and concerns. It was also intended to let her know I wanted her input and valued her opinion.

Mrs. Sabate's blood sugars were usually greater than 150, and she frequently needed sliding-scale insulin. Recognizing that her culture influenced her food choices, and knowing she was trying to control her diabetes, I offered help planning her meals so she could meet both these important needs. I helped her fill out the menu. I ordered a nutrition consult to provide coaching in making better food choices while still enjoying her native dishes. I emphasized the importance of proper blood-sugar monitoring and insulin-administration and the impact these measures had on her health. Mrs. Sabate agreed, and during her stay, her blood sugar became controlled such that she no longer needed regular sliding-scale insulin.

I was scheduled for a few days off and knew I wouldn't see Mrs. Sabate again before she was discharged, so I wished her the best at the end of my shift. But when I returned on Monday, I was surprised to see that Mrs. Sabate was still hospitalized. I was assigned to her. During report, I learned she had developed a wound complication; her incision had dehisced, and frequent dressing changes were necessary. When I entered her room, Mrs. Sabate was happy to see me.

The plan was for Mrs. Sabate to be discharged that day with visiting nurses for dressing changes. Prior to discharge, her doctor and I removed the dressing and noted that the wound edges hadn't approximated, and drainage persisted, which were signs that healing was not progressing. I was experienced in wound care and recognized that she'd need a vacuum assisted closure (VAC) dressing. Her physician and a wound specialist agreed, so the VAC was placed.

Mr. Sabate had been at home with their other children. When he arrived and learned what had transpired, he began to yell and blame staff. Usually in matters like this, the social worker would be paged to help, but due to Mr. Sabate's distrust of social work, I didn't think that would be a wise course. In spite of feeling somewhat intimidated and unsure, I sat with Mr. Sabate and spoke calmly as I explained that his wife's incision wasn't healing and a VAC dressing had been applied. I assured him that his wife's health was our highest priority. To my relief, his mood improved. It turned out it wasn't his wife's current situation that was weighing on him; it was what had transpired with the social worker prior to her delivery that was troubling him. He explained how the DCF workers were asking questions and coming to his home to observe how he cared for his children.

When Mr. Sabate spoke to the doctors, he vented his concerns again. I realized that although he appeared aggressive, even domineering, on the surface, on the inside he was a kind man seeking the best for his family in unfamiliar surroundings. I assured him again that our priority was to provide the best possible care to his wife. I became even more empathetic toward him, and a true trust developed between all of us.

From my attendance at cultural diversity programs, I knew that women were not viewed as equal to men in the Muslim culture, and their role often focused on raising children and caring for the family. During her extended time on the unit, while I was supporting her during breastfeeding, I mentioned the advantages of improving her English skills—how speaking and understanding English could help support her health and the health of her children. By this time Mrs. Sabate and I were close enough to joke about certain things. I kidded her about not wanting to see her back on the unit any time soon. She smiled and said, "Well, maybe one more time." Eventually, her wound healed, and she was able to go home. When she left, I thought it would be the last time I'd see her.

This past fall, one of my shifts began as usual, with report on my patients for the day. I got report on a 38-year-old woman who had delivered a healthy girl via repeat C-section. When I entered the patient's room, I was surprised to see it was Mrs. Sabate and her husband holding a new baby. It was certainly déjà vu.

Both Mr. and Mrs. Sabate were happy to see me and gave me a big smile and hug. I couldn't help noticing there was something different about Mrs. Sabate.

She had lost weight and appeared more vibrant than the last time I saw her. Her English had improved enough that I didn't have to call an interpreter. Mr. Sabate was much more relaxed, rocking in a chair with his newborn. I asked about the other children and he told me they were in school, doing well, and he was doing well at work.

Mr. Sabate brought up the DCF visits that had started during his wife's last hospitalization, but it wasn't in a negative way. He said it had actually been a positive experience. It had resulted in getting them access to resources to assist with the children's needs and finances. He again mentioned how happy he was to see a familiar face. When he left to check on the rest of the family, he said, "I know you'll take good care of her."

When he was gone, Mrs. Sabate said, "See how much more English I know." She told me that after her recovery from her previous C-section, she'd begun English classes at a school that offered drop-in child care. I was heartened to hear she had heeded my advice.

Throughout my interactions with Mrs. Sabate, I saw a dramatic difference in her. She made better food choices, and her blood sugar remained stable. I learned that she had used the educational materials the nutritionist and I had given her to make lifestyle changes. She was also using the diabetic clinic as a resource.

Another difference was that Mrs. Sabate left her room and ambulated in the hallway several times a day, pushing her daughter in her bassinet. During her previous stay she was reluctant to get out of bed, let alone leave her room. Before she'd had every excuse; now she displayed a new zeal. She had come a very long way.

Just before discharge, Mrs. Sabate thanked me for my patience, for educating her, and for offering emotional support. She said, "You're such a kind and caring person. I'm thankful you were my nurse." That statement has stayed with me and made me realize my impact as a nurse. How happy I am to have met and gotten to know Mrs. Sabate, her family, and her culture. She reaffirmed for me that I have chosen the right profession.

Commentary

Shauna's narrative again shows us the importance of clinicians entering the world of the patients and their families with openness to what they will see and hear. Shauna recognized that behind Mr. Sabate's anger was fear and worry, and she did not retreat from the emotion; instead, she stayed present and engaged. Her courage in that situation began to build the foundation of trust. Shauna's attention to the Sabates' culture informed her care and also served as a gateway into building the health of the family by empowering Mrs. Sabate. Like many nurses and clinicians, Shauna had not realized the impact she had on her patients; given what Mrs. Sabate told her, her influence on her patients and their families is great and long lasting.

Reflective Questions

- Mr. and Mrs. Sabate did not want the C-section based on their faith. What strategies might you use to help the family reevaluate their decision that was faith based?

- How might you shift your colleagues' perceptions of a patient or family member following an emotional outburst?

- Calling in DCF can tell a family, "We do not think you are good parents." How do you maintain a therapeutic relationship after something like that happens?

Opening the Door—#2

Susan Barisano, RN   **Practice level: Clinical Scholar**
Clinical Nurse, Post Anesthesia Care

One afternoon, I admitted Mr. Jameson, a 61-year-old-man who had come to our hospital from out of state for a partial laryngectomy and tracheostomy for laryngeal cancer. Mr. Jameson's surgical course was uneventful; he arrived in the PACU in stable condition. During my years as a nurse working in many critical care settings, I've cared for countless patients with tracheostomies, so I was comfortable initiating a plan of care for Mr. Jameson. I assessed his airway to ensure that he was oxygenating and ventilating adequately. He was hemodynamically stable. I assessed him for pain. He was still somnolent from the anesthesia, but when I asked if he was in pain he was able to indicate that he was not by shaking his head. I worked with the respiratory therapist to determine that Mr. Jameson's airway was clear, and we placed him on 40% oxygen with heated humidity via a trach mask. Satisfied with my postoperative assessment, I moved on to his communication needs.

Over the years, I've developed certain skills in assessing and managing complex airways and techniques to communicate with patients who are unable to speak. Patients with tracheostomies need to rely on staff's ability to lip-read, interpret gestures, or decipher handwritten notes. My goal was to ensure Mr. Jameson had a means of communication as he came out of anesthesia. I obtained a communication board, a pad of paper, and a pen for him. I provided him with a call light, and educated the operations associate about Mr. Jameson's inability to speak and the plan for communicating with him. I opened the curtain to his area so we could have visual access to Mr. Jameson during this immediate postoperative phase and he could signal us, if needed.

As time passed, and Mr. Jameson became more awake, he complained of increasing throat and neck pain. Laryngeal surgery doesn't typically cause a considerable amount of pain, but Mr. Jameson had been taking narcotics on occasion at home to control chronic lower-back pain. As a result, he had a higher than average pain-medication requirement. I collaborated with the PACU anesthesia and thoracic surgical teams to initiate a patient-controlled analgesia (PCA) for improved pain management and educated Mr. Jameson in the nuances of patient-controlled analgesia. Within a short period, Mr. Jameson and I were satisfied with the effects of the PCA.

As Mr. Jameson continued to recover from anesthesia, he became more aware of his surroundings. I stayed at his bedside, reassuring him and providing information about the surgery and plan of care. I began the process of educating him about the care and management of his tracheostomy, allowing myself ample time to be thorough. Because I've seen many patients with tracheostomies become frustrated or frightened by their inability to speak, I made sure that Mr. Jameson knew he could get the information he needed by writing his questions down. Mr. Jameson began conversing with me in writing but soon discovered that if he "spoke," he was easily understood, which made communication between us a little more natural.

Next, I set about locating Mr. Jameson's wife. Family members aren't often present in the PACU during the immediate postoperative phase, but I thought in this instance Mrs. Jameson's presence would be a comfort to her husband. And because Mr. Jameson had a new tracheostomy, I wanted him to have the company of his wife as he became accustomed to his situation. When Mrs. Jameson arrived, she had many questions and concerns but was happy to see her husband. I updated her on Mr. Jameson's progress and plan of care. She sat with him as he continued to recover, and Mr. Jameson appeared to rest more comfortably with his wife at his side.

I was informed that a bed would not become available for Mr. Jameson until later that evening. Staff on that unit wanted to situate him in a room close to the nurses' station, given that he had a new tracheostomy. I relayed this information to Mr. and Mrs. Jameson, and I encouraged Mrs. Jameson to return to the hotel, as it had been a very long day for both of them. To alleviate any anxiety she might have about leaving her husband, I provided her with phone numbers and information as to how she could stay in touch overnight by telephone. I suggested she return to the hospital in the morning, when she and Mr. Jameson would both be better rested.

Mrs. Jameson agreed and gathered her belongings. As she was getting ready to leave, she asked for help finding her way back to her hotel, which was several towns away from Boston. Her plan was to walk to the subway station, take the subway, then a bus, then walk the rest of the way to the hotel. She said she wasn't a "city girl" and had never taken public transportation. I could see she was nervous, and Mr. Jameson could see it, too. The idea of taking public transportation after dark in a strange city was daunting.

I consulted the case manager on-call to see if I could obtain a taxi voucher for Mrs. Jameson (something I had done on occasion when I worked in other settings, but I'd never needed it in the PACU). The case manager agreed with our concerns and arranged for a taxi voucher to be brought to the PACU. I gave it to Mrs. Jameson, and both she and Mr. Jameson were greatly relieved.

Before she left, I encouraged Mrs. Jameson to use the phone numbers I'd given her to check on her husband at any time throughout the night. I assured her that I'd call when her husband had been transferred to the unit and settled in his room. Then I asked one of our patient care associates to escort Mrs. Jameson to the taxi stand in front of the hospital, ensuring that all her transportation needs were being met.

In reflecting on the care I provided to Mr. Jameson, I feel I was able to attend not only to his clinical needs but also to the psychosocial needs of both Mr. Jameson and his wife. It's this ability to assist patients and family members in need and make a difference in their lives that truly guides my practice.

Commentary

In this rapidly changing environment, which requires constant vigilance to technology and the patients' response to interventions, Susan's narrative allows us to see the "big picture." In seeing that big picture, she immediately recognized the need to invite Mrs. Jameson to stay at her husband's side. Given the space constraints of the PACU setting and the concerns of the privacy of other patients, Susan could have faced push back from her colleagues, but her focus was on Mr. Jameson.

Susan recognized all that Mr. Jameson had gone through prior to meeting him—his cancer diagnosis, his inability to communicate easily, and the anxiety he was experiencing—and brought the couple together. Susan created a welcoming environment for Mrs. Jameson and noted that Mr. Jameson was calmer with his wife present.

Susan's concern for Mrs. Jameson to rest uncovered the fact that Mrs. Jameson had a very challenging journey as she returned to her hotel. Once again, Susan acted in her role as advocate—this time for Mrs. Jameson in securing a taxi voucher. Susan empathized with what Mrs. Jameson was facing and called upon past experience to reach out to the resource who could address this issue.

Reflective Questions

- How frequently do you address the psychosocial needs of patients and their family members? How do you work with physicians and other members of the team to see the whole patient?

- Families are not routinely brought into the PACU. What would you do if a colleague challenged your decision to have family members be with the patient?

- Family presence in the PACU is a major culture change for a staff/unit. What do you think can be done to encourage greater involvement of families in the PACU and other perioperative areas?

My Mother's Eyes

Donna Slicis, RN   **Practice level: Clinical Scholar**
Clinical Nurse, Cardiac Intensive Care

I do not know her. She is 86 years old. She was admitted to the Cardiac Intensive Care Unit during the day. It is the night shift. I am her nurse. It's 11:30 p.m. The day is ending, and this woman will not live to see another day. I do not know her.

I do not know him. He is her son. He has a looming presence. I watch him walk. Pacing, to and from the secretaries' desk. He seeks information about his mother. Her nurse is in report. I am told he is the oldest of eight children; he is 65 years old. I do not know him.

I know his concern. It is an all-consuming concern. He is the leader of his family and friends. There are more than 40 who follow this man. All grieving the dying woman, all led by this worried man, whom I don't know.

Where to begin is obvious only to me. Start to know this dying woman. The family would want answers that I would not have if I went to them first. The woman is intubated, sedated, and in cardiogenic shock. Her bed's headboard is filled with small pumps, each willing her blood pressure a little higher and her heart to beat a little stronger. She is on 100% oxygen but still has poor blood gases. She appears comfortable on her current doses of sedatives and analgesics. She appears to be asleep, unresponsive to verbal stimuli, but her eyes are open. I try to shut her eyes; they do not shut. I try keeping them shut with eye lubricant; they do not shut. I try to gently hold them shut. They open.

Other than her open eyes, she appears comfortable. She is clean and neat. The room is orderly and tidy. I comb her hair. I fix her pillows and adjust her sheets. I turn down the lights. I place tissue boxes around the room. I lower her bed. I write down her current vital signs, my assessment, medication names, and drip rate.

There will be no changing of her drips; they are not working. Her heart is failing, and there is nothing that will change that. Helping her look comfortable is a difficult task. She is edematous, blue, and cold and covered with tubes and wires. She looks like she is dying. Cindy, our secretary for the night, calls the family into the unit at my request; I meet the family outside of her room.

"Hello, my name is Donna, and I will be her nurse for the night. She has many tubes and wires attached to her right now, but she appears comfortable. I do not believe she will live through the night. She is on several different medications, and her heart continues to fail. After you see her, I'll have the doctor come in and give you an update. Before you go in, there is something you should know. I could not get her eyes to close. Her eyes are open, but she appears to be sleeping and comfortable."

I felt as though my frustration would engulf me. This large group of people loved this woman. I could not make her hand warm to the touch. I could not make her skin color pink and healthy. I could not make her well. Why couldn't I just get her eyes to close? She would then, at least, appear to be sleeping, restfully and peacefully.

Laughter. Laughing from the group, but not the concerned man. The entire group was finding something I said amusing. "My mother always slept with her eyes open," said one. "She had eight kids; how else do you think she kept track of them?" said another. "She would scare our friends when we were younger," said another. Now, more laughter as they entered the room of the dying woman they loved.

There were no questions from them. The concerned son did not enter the room. He stood alone outside the room. He did not find relief from anxiety in laughter; he was still worried. He needed a nurse, yet he was hours away from sharing his feelings and minutes away from it not mattering.

"Tell me how you're feeling," I said to the son. Then came what I least expected from him—tears, tears, and more tears. I had no tissues ready for this, and leaving to find some was not an option. Through his tears he began: He was the man who took his mother earlier in the week to make her own funeral arrangements. His mother wanted simple arrangements and wanted to ensure that things were done her way. I listened. His mother was loved by many; she was a good mother; she was involved with her church; and she was a friend to many. I listened. His mother had been well the day before she made her funeral arrangements. Did he miss something? I listened. His mother had come to the hospital to die. Her son, the eldest, asked her to live. When she agreed, her long-standing do-not-resuscitate order was rescinded. His mother had spent the day in the cardiac catheterization lab. Procedure after procedure and still her heart was failing. I listened.

Now I knew him. His worry started when he asked his mother to take a chance on life and it didn't work. He wanted the do-not-resuscitate order reinstated.

After a long discussion with him and the rest of the family, it was clear that no one wanted this woman to experience chest compressions, defibrillation, or any other aggressive heroics. The resident on-call was extremely supportive and also understood that the family—and especially the eldest son—needed their mother protected against medical intervention that would only extend the inevitability of death, not prevent it.

Her cardiologist would have preferred that all decisions wait until morning, but this decision could not wait, and the family was in need of control. The friends and family were given control, and the eldest son went into the room to face the open eyes of his mother.

My peers made coffee for this extremely large family. They helped find chairs, telephones, and blankets. They helped me with anything I needed and with some things I didn't even know I needed. No one questioned the family members' wandering; they were free to come and go, in and out of the unit.

Wrapped in blankets, they gathered by her bedside—sometimes all of them, sometimes some of them. My focus was on the comfort of the woman and facilitating the grieving for her family and friends.

The change in focus, to that of comfort, enabled grieving to be fostered. I prepared them for what dying would look like. I encouraged them to share thoughts and regrets. I encouraged them to let go of what could not be changed.

Now that the woman was actively dying, I asked the family to teach me about this woman. Stories were told—some with tears, others with laughter. Her minister arrived. Songs were sung. Prayers were said. Grieving began. Now I knew this family, and I knew this woman, Norma. Then she dies. Eyes open.

One by one, each of Norma's family left the room, all sharing their love of Norma with me. All taking their time to express their relief and gratitude that Norma's death went so well. A good death.

All that remained was Norma's son, the eldest. All the worry was gone. "Donna," he said, as he walked toward me, "I closed my mother's eyes for you." The eldest son was nursing the nurse, and how I now wished that his mother's eyes were open to see this.

Commentary

With the statement, "Tell me how you're feeling," Donna allowed Norma's son the opportunity to grieve. It was a risk to ask this question; it is much easier to assume we know someone is worried or sad or upset. Experts take such risks. Donna does not assume she knows why he is concerned; she just knows that his feelings are preventing him from being with his mother and family. The wisdom of this narrative is that we need to be more curious about others to wonder, ask questions, and then listen to what they have to say.

Reflective Questions

- Do you think it takes courage to ask Norma's son to share his feelings? How do you find such courage?

- Donna's statement that she could not close their mother's eyes allowed Norma's children the opportunity to reminisce and begin to grieve. Is the process of reminiscing about a loved one an important step for a family prior to a death? How do you guide a family as they begin this process?

- Donna pays great attention to how Norma's room looks and where chairs and tissues are, and that coffee is brought to the family; these are wonderful caring practices. How do you develop caring practices in yourself, in your colleagues, and in the culture of a unit?

When Public Policy Becomes Personal

Julie Berrett-Abebe, LICSW   **Practice level: Clinical Scholar**
Clinical Social Worker, Oncology

In my work as an oncology social worker, I've been fortunate to collaborate with skilled and compassionate multidisciplinary colleagues who have shared much with me about the exciting developments in the breast cancer world. Many of these advances relate to personalized medicine and targeted therapies. I've learned that prognoses both for women with earlier stage breast cancer as well as women with metastatic breast cancer have improved as they receive treatments targeted specifically to "their cancer." However, the psychosocial impact of receiving longer-term treatments and living with a chronic illness is often profound. Particularly in our current economy, financial and employment-related concerns are causing distress for many patients, even those whom we typically think of as financially secure. In this narrative, I describe a short-term counseling intervention for a newly diagnosed breast cancer patient, focusing on clinical interventions related to employment-related concerns and anxiety.

Gail is a 39-year-old woman with no family history of breast cancer who was diagnosed with an invasive cancer. Immediately upon her diagnosis, she asked to speak with a social worker to address anxiety related to her diagnosis, worries for the future, and concerns about employment. Gail lives with her husband and two young daughters in a Boston suburb. She is a vice president of a local company and provides a large share of her family's income. Gail met with a therapist in the past to work through bereavement following significant losses.

My initial meeting with Gail took place one week after her diagnosis. Although still experiencing shock regarding her diagnosis, Gail decided that she wanted to treat the cancer "aggressively" and had made plans to have bilateral mastectomies with reconstruction right away. Gail came to my office with a list of questions and concerns. "I can't stop thinking about dying in the future from cancer… how do people cope with this?" "How much information should I share with my children?" "My father died unexpectedly last year; what's the best way to talk to my mother and siblings about my illness without making them frightened?" "I'm in a fairly new position at work, and I want to maintain a balance between transparency and privacy. I also don't want to be fired or have others think I can't do my job. How can I work through this?"

In our first counseling session, I provided several interventions: I listened as Gail shared her narrative. I normalized shock and anxiety related to diagnosis and provided suggestions of strategies to manage anxiety (distraction for anxiety related to testing and diaphragmatic breathing, relaxation, and Cognitive Behavioral Therapy (CBT) techniques to address anxiety related to cancer). I provided education about sharing information with children. I also provided information about programs such as the Family and Medical Leave Act (FMLA) and short-term disability as well as suggestions for gathering information from Human Resources at work. I helped Gail to consider who at work needed to know immediately about her diagnosis and what decisions she needed to make right away. She wrote an initial plan for managing work concerns as we spoke.

Gail called me later in the week to work through writing two scripts: one for sharing information about her diagnosis with her employer (and stating her preference that this information not be shared with other employees) and one for sharing information about her diagnosis with her family. Gail expressed great appreciation for my expertise related to illness and employment, my knowledge of good communication skills, and my ability to help her process her own feelings and concerns.

Gail and I had a few other face-to-face meetings after her surgery. Gail's surgery was quite extensive and required a lengthy recovery period. She also completed several rounds of chemotherapy after healing from surgery. When her chemotherapy treatments were complete, I helped Gail craft a plan for her return to work, prioritizing good communication with her employer and a focus on her own self-care. Gail worked from home for several weeks; when she finally returned to work full time, Gail stated that she was "ready." Gail and I also addressed her anxiety about cancer recurrence (which was also an impediment to her focusing on work and family responsibilities). We did a piece of counseling work together, and I provided referrals for longer-term counseling in the community as needed.

Gail often expressed appreciation for my counseling skills, oncology experience, and policy knowledge, stating that they made a difference in helping her cope with her illness. It was gratifying to work with someone who was so motivated and made good use of my role on the multidisciplinary healthcare team.

My work with Gail caused me to think about the United States' public policy related to work and disability. The United States does not have (and never has had) a comprehensive policy for paid time off for disability, child care, or illness. I am inspired by Gail and countless other women like her to pursue the issues of employment and paid time off as they relate to cancer as an area of research during my social work doctoral studies. I have also begun to reflect upon how social workers might be able to better articulate the support we provide to patients regarding employment and cancer. Often, team members think about social workers providing financial support resources to those in need (and this is indeed an important role), but I think more broadly we are experts in helping people manage relationships (those in the workplace being no exception). This will become an ever more important issue as we have the good fortune to see the number of cancer survivors increase with each passing year.

Commentary

Like so many people who receive a cancer diagnosis, Gail's life was changed in an instant. And her diagnosis affected not only Gail, but also her family, her company, and her colleagues. Julie's experience with caring for patients and families in similar situations was a source of substantive guidance and information as well as comfort and solace. Her strategies for coping with anxiety, reigning in fear, and "getting on with life" were key to Gail's ability to develop self-reliance and self-knowledge on her own needs. Not only did Julie focus her expertise on Gail's needs, but also she saw this situation as part of a larger discourse on how our nation supports its citizens in times of illness and disability.

Reflective Questions

- Gail struggled with a very common question for patients, "How do I live my life with a diagnosis of cancer?" How do you help break down this incredibly complex question and all the meaning this question holds?

- In this narrative, Julie used CBT with Gail. How do you know when CBT will be an effective intervention for a patient?

- As clinicians, what do you think we can do to begin a conversation on this public policy question?

Summary

In this chapter you read narratives on a theme that is central to why clinicians chose their profession—the desire to care for and help patients. As simple as that desire is, forming a relationship with patients requires skill, insight, and experience. The less experienced may consider forming a therapeutic relationship as "liking" the patient. With greater experience, the clinician moves from defining the therapeutic relationship as a personal "liking" to knowing the patient and forging a relationship based on achieving the best outcomes for the patient in an open, nonjudgmental manner.

We believe that guiding clinicians to reflect on this theme allows for not only their professional growth but also their ability to strengthen their practice in the other themes of practice—clinical knowledge and decision-making, team-work and collaboration, and, in Occupational Therapy and Physical Therapy, movement.

Chapter 3
Theme of Practice: Clinical Knowledge and Decision-Making

The understanding attained through formal and experiential learning

---

IN THIS CHAPTER

- Putting the pieces together
- Redefining success
- Running toward a goal
- Remembering to breathe
- Empowering the patient

The Importance of Clinical Knowledge and Decision-Making

It was not surprising that clinical knowledge and decision-making was a theme found throughout the narratives of clinicians in Nursing and Patient Care Services. Clinicians care for acutely ill patients utilizing cutting-edge technology, complex treatment, and therapies on a daily basis. The patients require clinicians whose practice is current and evidence based and who are able to synthesize large amounts of knowledge.

The theoretical foundation for the Clinical Recognition Program at Massachusetts General Hospital is the Dreyfus brothers' work on skill acquisition (Dreyfus & Dreyfus, 1986). As described in Chapter 1, skill acquisition is the development of skilled "know-how." Skilled know-how is essential in any practice discipline. It is what enables a clinician to deliver care to a patient, titrate a medication, or know when a patient is ready for the next step in his or her recovery. Skilled know-how is not innate; it has to be learned through trial and error or guided by someone with experience. Clinicians acquire and maintain skilled know-how through practice. Clinical practice requires both theoretical "knowing that" and experiential "knowing how."

The knowledge that new clinicians bring as they begin their careers comes mostly from textbooks and lectures, as well as limited exposure to patients. This knowledge enables them to order and structure their clinical assignments and to pass licensing exams. But when these new clinicians gain exposure to the realities of practice, they often feel unprepared and overwhelmed. For experienced clinicians, theoretical knowledge is informed by their involvement in the care of patients and families.

EXPERIENCE DEFINED

At MGH, experience is not defined by the mere passage of time. Rather, we embrace Patricia Benner's definition: "It is the refinement of preconceived notions and theory by encountering many actual practical situations that add nuances or shades of differences to theory."

Narratives—Entry Level of Practice

The narratives of clinicians at the advanced beginner or Entry level of practice reflect the work of integrating theoretical knowledge with the actual experience of caring for patients. At this stage narratives often read like a list of tasks and procedures that were accomplished without a true understanding of the "big picture."

Narratives—Clinician Level of Practice

With continued experience the clinician develops a mastery of the technical skills and becomes increasingly aware of similarities in the patient's condition and responses, which allow the clinician to anticipate and plan. Narratives at this stage reflect greater understanding of the patients' condition as well as the limitations clinicians recognize in their own skill, knowledge, and ability.

Narratives—Advanced Clinician Level of Practice

At the proficient or Advanced Clinician level, the clinicians' narratives reflect their engagement and confidence in the clinical situation. They spend less time on analysis; rather, they often describe as seeing or knowing what is important in the situation and then doing what is needed to accomplish the task. At this level, the clinician exhibits an increasing comfort in taking "clinically sound risks." Experience allows the clinicians to move from a clinical situation, where there is a long list of "possibilities," to a more concise list of "probabilities" where past actions have been successful, and so they intervene. This comfort in reading the situation allows the Advanced Clinician to more effectively and efficiently manage the situation.

Narratives—Clinical Scholar Level of Practice

At the expert or Clinical Scholar level, the clinicians' clinical knowledge and decision-making process often disappear in the narrative. The clinician no longer goes through the lengthy analysis and processing that's evident in the less-experienced clinician's description of the situation. Rather, Clinical Scholars intuitively know and understand what is happening in the situation and what should be done—they are at one with the situation. Their clinically sound risk-taking is consistent and fluid, the solution or intervention seeming to just appear. This allows them to truly focus on the issue and concerns at hand.

The narratives that follow describe the clinical knowledge and decision-making theme of practice across the six disciplines and across the four levels of expertise, as described in Chapter 1. The unbundling through reflective questions, which follows a brief commentary on the narrative, allows you to reflect on your own practice or that of a colleague.

Tea for Four

Danuza "Danny" Nunn, SLP-CCC
Speech-Language Pathologist

Practice level: Clinician

Mary was a 90-year-old woman with a history of advanced dementia. She was admitted due to acute changes in her mental status accompanied by pneumonia. Speech-Language Pathology was consulted to evaluate her ability to swallow and her risk for aspiration. She had been in the hospital for nearly a week, her stay complicated by her worsening mental status and concern about failure to thrive.

Mary had two devoted daughters who were by her side every day. They were very concerned they may have inadvertently done something to contribute to their mom's aspiration. They were eager to find out whether they needed to change her diet or learn a new way to feed her. She had been prescribed pureed and honey-thick liquids but was either refusing to eat or was too somnolent to be fed. The daughters reported that at home she'd had a good appetite and loved to eat.

Despite her advanced dementia prior to admission, she'd been able to feed herself. They hadn't noticed any coughing or choking, no recent vomiting, and no recent changes in her weight. They did note that she had become more somnolent and sounded congested, and she hadn't eaten or drunk anything that day before being admitted. Mary had spiked a fever before being brought to the hospital.

Mary's daughters reported that since being admitted, she wasn't "behaving like herself," appearing agitated and/or lethargic. Because of her refusal to eat and drink, she was placed on IV fluids and IV antibiotics. The team had tried to place a nasogastric tube, but Mary was too agitated to tolerate it.

Mary was fidgety. When her daughters left the room, she would try to remove her IV (which she managed to do three times). She experienced increased agitation at night, requiring sedation, which made her somnolent the next day, affecting her ability to participate in her care. She had been able to walk at home but hadn't been out of bed since being admitted.

My initial session with Mary was spent gathering information, trying to learn as much as I could about her likes, dislikes, and typical routine. We discussed how just being in the hospital can cause behavioral changes—being in an unfamiliar environment, having her routine disrupted, taking medications, and being exposed to unfamiliar people and situations.

Mary's daughters were concerned that she was still refusing to eat or drink. I suggested we try offering her some familiar foods and let her try to eat on her own (instead of feeding her). The daughters were concerned because the doctors had mentioned that their mom had aspirated. I still had hope that her pneumonia might be unrelated to the aspiration. I reminded them that Mary had been independent with feeding, hadn't lost weight prior to admission, and hadn't had any prior pulmonary infections. She hadn't shown any typical signs of aspiration or feeding issues usually observed with dementia patients (like pocketing, decreased chewing, or forgetting to swallow).

I could see they were distraught and afraid that Mary might decline further, or worse, that she might not be able to eat anymore. I reminded them I'd been consulted to make sure that Mary was able to eat and drink safely and evaluate whether she was aspirating or not. I assured them that I wouldn't do anything to harm or aggravate their mother. I felt the best way to proceed was to allow her to do what she did naturally.

I had learned that Mary loved cookies and tea. So instead of conducting a typical evaluation where I would observe Mary eating and drinking, I arranged a little "tea party." We set up a table beside her bed, complete with cookies and teacups. I invited Mary's daughters to join in and partake of the snacks. Mary, who hadn't eaten anything, hesitated briefly, but when she saw her daughters grab a cookie, she promptly reached for one, too.

The tension in the room evaporated as we all laughed. Mary ate the whole cookie with no difficulty, and then asked for ice cream. Her daughter's were shocked at the change in Mary's behavior. I reminded them that Mary had presented with no signs of deterioration of her feeding skills or aspiration. It was just that being hospitalized was a challenge for her.

I shared that both of my grandmothers had suffered from dementia, and their abilities had deteriorated when they were hospitalized. This has made me more attuned to the impact of care on patients with dementia. I explained that Mary's abilities would probably fluctuate during her hospitalization, and it would be important to try to normalize her routine as much as possible. Identifying factors that led to agitation would be helpful. I acknowledged how lucky Mary was to have daughters who were so devoted to her and how important they were in assisting us in caring for her.

I stressed the importance of minimizing things that might further disrupt her routine and/or agitate her. I advised them that our geriatric team and/or psychiatric CNS teams would be good resources in this area.

It was very rewarding to come in the next day and see everyone working together. The teams had spoken with some resources and were given some very helpful suggestions. Nurses on the unit were key in implementing those suggestions. Mary's bed was moved closer to the window so she could tell whether it was day or night. They didn't check her vital signs at night so she could get a good night's sleep. Mary was assigned the same nurses and patient care associates for consistency and to increase her familiarity with her caregivers. Staff posted a list of her favorite foods so that they could be requested for her. She was able to wear some of her own clothes, and her daughters brought in a few things from home to make the room more familiar.

Mary's agitation was managed with de-escalation techniques, such as looking at family pictures, playing cards, and listening to music.

She was upgraded to a regular diet with thin liquids, and she was able to eat uneventfully.

Mary was discharged a few days later, when she was able to be transitioned to oral antibiotics.

Although I know part of Mary's improvement was due to antibiotics and the eventual resolution of her pneumonia, I felt honored to be involved in her care. I think sharing my personal and professional experience with dementia had an impact on Mary's outcome, and tapping into the pool of expertise and resources that are available was key. They say it takes a village, and, in this case, it certainly did.

Commentary

What did you think of when you heard the patient was a 90-year-old with advanced dementia and a question of aspiration pneumonia? She was also not eating, agitated, and pulling out her IVs. Most likely, you would have implemented many of the interventions recounted in this narrative.

Danny entered the room and paused. She listened to Mary's daughters tell her who their mother is. Danny entertained the possibility that the pneumonia was not related to aspiration and used her knowledge and experience to take a clinically sound risk by having a tea party. She replicated, as best she could, an afternoon tea with Mary's daughters. Surrounded by family and familiar food and drink, the Mary that her daughters know and love reappeared.

Reflective Questions

- Danny developed an interdisciplinary plan to bring resources and support to Mary while she was hospitalized. How would you accomplish a plan such as this?

- What if the team feels your plan of care is too risky? What would you do?

- Danny shared personal information with Mary's daughters about her personal experience with dementia. How do you make the decision when and how to share personal information with a patient and/or family?

Learning to Relax

Christine Carifio, OTR/L   **Practice level: Clinician**
Occupational Therapist

I first met John on a General Medical Unit. He was a 69-year-old man with a history of hepatitis C, stage IV non-small-cell lung cancer, and epilepsy. He presented with possible pneumonia and urinary tract infection. He had an unsteady gait and looked much older than his age.

John was sitting up in bed eating breakfast with his wife, Judy, at his bedside. The first thing I noticed was the physical shaking as he attempted to feed himself. His entire body shook, making the eating process very challenging, but he was determined to try to feed himself with no assistance. John shared with me that he wasn't sure of the origin of the tremors, but he knew they got worse with increased anxiety. During my evaluation, John did appear anxious, frazzled, and overwhelmed.

I explained the role of occupational therapists to John and how we try to help individuals regain the means and ability to perform everyday activities. But given what I had learned in my chart review, the time I'd spent on the Psychiatric Unit, and my observations of his apparent anxiety, I decided to add that occupational therapists also facilitate coping strategies. This could help John manage his anxiety so he'd have a better opportunity to participate more fully in his daily roles and routines.

After explaining the idea of managing anxiety versus strictly helping with physical impairments, both John's and his wife's interest were piqued. Both agreed, "That's something we're really interested in."

After my initial evaluation, John's wife followed me out of the room with many questions about his anxiety. She told me she believed anxiety was the root of his poor function. She shared that they had recently moved out of a home where John had lived for 30 years and how the event had triggered extreme anxiety. Prior to this hospital admission, John had been a fairly independent man. He was retired and independent with basic activities of daily living (IADLs). However, now that they had moved, he received assistance from her for most

IADLs, and she reported that he had started drinking more in an effort to ease the anxiety.

My "mental-health brain" perked up. What she was describing were the sort of questions I asked patients on the Psychiatric Unit. I wanted to help John and his wife not only with his physical disabilities, but also from a mental-health perspective. I consulted his chart to ensure that Psychiatry was following John. I found that they were prescribing several medications for anxiety and agitation, as needed.

During my next session with John, I began by introducing relaxation strategies in hopes that after trying them, he'd calm down enough to be able to participate in more activities of daily living. John demonstrated insight into his anxiety and seemed interested in hearing about sensory strategies, deep breathing, and other relaxation techniques. I gave him a ball to squeeze, which he immediately clung to. And I had him practice deep-breathing exercises while supine in bed. After completing just a few relaxation exercises, it was amazing how much more we were able to accomplish.

The shaking was still significant, but John was motivated for therapy. We were able to do edge-of-bed activities and lower-body dressing with assistance. I noticed that when John performed upper-extremity exercises, his shakiness decreased dramatically—which again brought me back to my time on the Psychiatric Unit and reminded me how repetitive-movement activities can be calming. And here I was seeing it in action on a medical unit.

I left John with a number of sensory objects and explained how he could use each of them and what they would do for him with the hope that he would carry these strategies over when I left. After our session, I looked back at the most recent psychiatry follow-up note in John's chart and one suggestion was, "Consider occupational therapy for sensory strategies." It looked like we were all on the same page.

Several days later, I met John for our second session. The first words out of his mouth were, "I was hoping you'd come back. I broke my squeeze ball!"

Again, I noticed an improvement with John's function after participating in relaxation strategies. And he reported that he enjoyed the candy I had provided (for oral stimulation) and wanted more. When I asked why he liked the candy, he said, "It helps me focus."

During this session, we were able to complete full-body bathing and dressing at the bedside and toileting using a commode—again progressing more than we had in the prior session and with me providing less assistance. The combination of medications to manage his anxiety, relaxation and coping strategies prior to activity, and participation in meaningful activities was working.

According to John's nurse and chart, the plan was for John to be discharged to a rehabilitation facility the next day with outpatient psychiatric follow-up.

Since then, I've learned that John is doing well at rehab, walking with a walker, and "doing better than when he came in." I felt that my experience with both mental health and physical disabilities served John's needs appropriately and effectively during his time on the medical unit. I hope to continue to employ sensory and coping strategies for improved function and participation in meaningful activities whenever the opportunity arises.

Commentary

Christine quickly recognized that John's symptoms had a strong psychological component, so she developed a holistic plan to encompass all of his symptoms, not just the physical ones. By partnering with John and his wife, they entered into a trusting, supportive relationship. This empowered Christine to draw on her experience and creativity and explore alternative strategies to meet John's needs. These strategies are applicable to many areas of practice as a way to engage and assist patients in coping with stress and anxiety.

Reflective Questions

- To help their patients, clinicians may facilitate coping strategies. How can you determine when patients would be open to looking at the psychological aspect of their conditions given their presenting physical symptoms?

- How does anxiety affect a patient's ability to heal? Do you consider a patient's anxiety in your care for that patient?

- The use of sensory interventions is an intervention that was very helpful to John. How would you go about assessing which sensory intervention is best for a particular patient?

Rethinking the Goal

Heidi Cheerman, PT   **Practice level: Advanced Clinician**
Physical Therapist

Having worked with patients with chronic neurological disorders for the past 9 years, I continue to be amazed at their ability to adapt and function under the most challenging conditions. In the acute-care setting, clinicians must be able to understand and build a rapport with patients in a very short period of time, often within a single treatment session. That means gathering, synthesizing, and integrating the most pertinent data to make effective clinical decisions on treatment approaches and recommendations.

Mr. Ortiz was a 48-year-old man with a history of multiple sclerosis (MS) and spastic paraparesis; he was admitted to MGH for management of varicella zoster (a herpes virus). Due to this infection he experienced generalized weakness prior to being admitted, which affected his functional mobility. The day he was admitted, his status had declined to the point that he could barely sit on the edge of his bed. In fact, he had fallen at home while attempting to transfer to his wheelchair.

Mr. Ortiz had experienced a steady decline in functional mobility over the last few years. Three years prior to admission he was walking independently. With the progressive nature of his disease, at the time of his admission he was spending most of his time in his wheelchair. He had maintained a strong sense of determination, which had allowed him to lead an independent life and be a supportive husband to his wife of 11 years.

In reviewing his chart, I noticed Mr. Ortiz had experienced a number of falls while at home over the last 2 years. During my interview with him, Mr. Ortiz explained that the falls occurred most often when transferring from his wheelchair to his bed (which is 3'2" high). My initial judgment was that Mr. Ortiz lacked insight into his functional limitations. Cognitive deficits are common in patients with MS, and, given his frequent falls, my thinking was that he probably shouldn't be left at home alone. Experience told me that I needed additional data in order to form an accurate impression.

During my initial evaluation, Mr. Ortiz was very positive and outgoing and exhibited a good sense of humor. One member of the team interpreted Mr. Ortiz's jokes as not taking his situation seriously. But through further observation, I came to understand that his reliance on humor was a coping strategy; it enabled him to deal with the stress of his current condition and the challenges of what had been a very difficult life.

Mr. Ortiz lived in a one-story, ramp-accessible home equipped with grab bars in the bathroom, a shower chair and a commode, a customized wheelchair, and a rolling walker for transfers. He was able to perform activities of daily living while his wife was at work, and she assisted him with laundry, grocery shopping, and other activities. His exam revealed decreased activity tolerance; postural control deficits; increased bilateral, lower-extremity tone; strength and motor control deficits; and range-of-motion deficits.

After being in bed for 4 days during this admission, Mr. Ortiz needed moderate assistance to sit on the edge of bed. When I removed my hand he initially lost his balance but recovered with internal feedback. Evaluating Mr. Ortiz's ability to transfer from the bed to the chair was a priority during this initial evaluation and critical to constructing a plan of care and recommendations for discharge.

I decided to set up a transfer that simulated Mr. Ortiz's home environment. I set his hospital bed to 3' high (neither foot able to reach the floor while sitting on the bed) and took into account his impairments and history of falling. I found myself doubting the safety of the plan, but Mr. Ortiz assured me he felt "100% confident" he could do it (based on doing it at home every day). I decided it was a sound clinical risk. To ensure his safety, I padded the floor around his bed and called his nurse and a patient care associate to help. He performed his transfer with moderate assistance, his movements resembling that of a patient with partial paralysis (i.e., depending on upper-body strength for mobility).

I brought up the idea of a short inpatient rehabilitation stay with Mr. Ortiz, but he was adamant that he wanted to go home, saying, "I just need to increase my mobility, and I'll get it back quickly. I know my body."

I called Mrs. Ortiz after the session, and she shared her concern about his "coming home in this condition." She had developmental issues that affected her short-term memory and problem-solving abilities. She also experienced anxiety in new situations. She expressed concern that if Mr. Ortiz went to rehab, "He might never come home." She agreed to come in the next day to discuss and observe her husband's status.

Prior to our session the next day, in order to gain more insight into Mr. Ortiz's care, I consulted with the physician who had been following his case over the past 5 years at the MS Clinic. I expressed my concern about his going home and my rationale for an acute inpatient rehabilitation stay. The physician felt strongly that it would be in Mr. Ortiz's best interest to be discharged home, citing the resources he had in place, his history of functioning well at home before, his history of depression, and the psychological stress of not being able to support his wife.

After my session with Mr. Ortiz and his wife, I had a greater understanding of their situation and was determined to find a solution for Mr. Ortiz to discharge home safely. Taking into account their concerns and Mr. Ortiz's goals, his physician's opinion, his home setup, and his functional abilities, I felt confident that Mr. Ortiz would function well if discharged home. Later that evening, I researched additional resources for Mr. Ortiz and his wife to support a successful discharge. Knowing the progression of MS and anticipating continued decline, I gathered information on home, self-transfer lift systems.

With continued PT intervention, Mr. Ortiz was able to safely and independently transfer to a level surface using a slide board. I coordinated with the case manager to have a hospital bed delivered to Mr. Ortiz's home to enable him to perform bed-to-wheelchair transfers at home with greater ease.

Many layers of complexity need to be peeled back to have a complete understanding of patients' needs. Mr. Ortiz was an example of how recommendations we initially think are in the best interest of our patients may not actually be optimal. By listening to Mr. Ortiz, his wife, and his physician of long standing, I was confident in my clinical decision to advocate for his discharge home. By digging beneath the surface, I was able to find additional resources for Mr. Ortiz. As I continue to move forward in my practice, Mr. Ortiz serves as a reminder that clinical decision-making is not a clear-cut process.

I ran into Mr. Ortiz's wife recently and heard he's functioning well at home. I felt further assured that the plan we put in place for him was working, which gave me a great sense of happiness for him and his wife.

Commentary

Flexibility, active listening, and an open mind: three key qualities in the delivery of patient- and family-centered care. Heidi skillfully assessed Mr. Ortiz's functional abilities and limitations, even simulating his home environment to ensure his safety. Heidi was thorough and persistent in creating a discharge plan that was clinically sound and met the unique needs of the patient and his wife. Perhaps most important, she left herself open to all options, driven not by the need to be right, but by the desire to do what was best for Mr. Ortiz.

Reflective Questions

- Flexibility, active listening, and an open mind are three key qualities in the delivery of patient- and family-centered care. How well do you exhibit these qualities? Can you give examples? In what ways can you improve in these three areas?

- Have you been in a situation where you could not support a discharge or treatment plan? What did you do?

- Mrs. Ortiz was concerned not only about her husband returning home, but also what would happen if he went to rehab. How do you support family members like Mrs. Ortiz through a difficult time such as the one described?

Red Flags

Theodora Abbenante, RN   **Practice level: Advanced Clinician**
Clinical Nurse, Vascular Surgery

As a staff nurse on a Vascular Surgical Unit over the past 10 years, I continue to be humbled by the complexity of our patient population. Our patients' multiple co-morbidities and chronic disease processes demand strong clinical skills and judgment that have driven my pursuit to stay knowledgeable in my practice. Just when I think I've seen it all, I encounter a patient or situation that demands a new perspective.

Mrs. Montgomery was an 82-year-old woman who had undergone a carotid endarterectomy. She had a past medical history complicated by diabetes, hypertension, coronary artery disease requiring bypass surgery, and an ejection fraction of 56%. As with any post-surgical carotid patient, complications can include stroke, reperfusion syndrome, hematoma further compromising the patient's airway, and hemodynamic instability with acute changes in blood pressure or heart rate. Mrs. Montgomery's age, past medical history, and ejection fraction increased these risks. I approached her care the way I do all my patients: I tried to arm myself with as much background information as I could from the patient's record and made sure I got all my questions answered during report from the Post-Acute Care Unit (PACU) nurse.

Right from the start of my telephone report with the PACU nurse, alarms were going off in my head. Combined with what I'd learned about Mrs. Montgomery's history, her intra-operative and PACU presentation suggested a high potential for complications. Mrs. Montgomery had had an episode of significant bradycardia during her surgery and was having difficulty weaning from the ventilator. I was told she had a history of pre-op heart rate in the 50s, and she was now stable and doing fine. Her heart rate, though low with dips into the 40s, was deemed her baseline. Immediately, I noted a downward trend in the numbers between intra-op and PACU vital signs. Given her age and history, there were red flags everywhere. I put the nurse on hold and shared my concerns with the resident, who felt Mrs. Montgomery was at her baseline low heart rate and stable for transfer. The resident didn't think the numbers were cause for alarm or feel a need to keep her in recovery any longer.

I felt uneasy with the clinical profile I was seeing and decided the best thing to do was be ready to handle any changes that happened when Mrs. Montgomery arrived. My first order of business was to establish a thorough physical baseline and empower myself with information about Mrs. Montgomery. I thought about her risk of flash pulmonary edema given her fluid status in the setting of her cardiac history, the risk of change in mental status given her episodes of hypotension, and the risk of acute arrhythmia as a result of all of the above. I was already on alert that we were overlooking her overall trends and chalking it up to a momentary episode of hypotension and a baseline low heart rate. According to the surgeons, she was stable. In the past, that would have given me comfort, but the nurse I am today finds comfort in my own clinical judgment, and I was not feeling comfortable.

As resource nurse, I notified staff that I was worried about the patient coming up from the PACU and if they needed me, I'd be with Mrs. Montgomery for a while after she arrived.

Mrs. Montgomery arrived, and I was happy to note she was alert and oriented; she was a very pleasant 82-year-old woman. Her systolic blood pressure was in the 90s; her heart rate in the 40–50s with occasional dips into the 30s with frequent ectopy. I took extra care in assessing her lungs as soon as she arrived and placed her on a cardiac monitor. I checked her blood pressure in both arms manually to rule out questions that might later arise. I kept a close watch on her heart rate and made frequent blood pressure checks. Her pressure quickly trended down to the 80s. I reconsidered her estimated blood loss, risk of bleeding, and fluid balance; I couldn't explain this drop, but I was confident that out of the PACU setting and without pressors she was slowly trending toward an unstable state. Knowing she'd had an acute episode intra-operatively, I was concerned we were heading in the wrong direction.

I quickly notified the team of the clinical profile I had compiled along with Mrs. Montgomery's current blood pressure. They weren't concerned and said they'd be in to see her in a few minutes during rounds. When they arrived, they acknowledged the low heart rate and blood pressure but felt that in the setting of her mental status and a pre-established baseline of low heart rate, she was stable. At this point, the words "baseline" and "stable" were becoming very frustrating. It seemed as though the team was making broad assumptions, and I wasn't being heard. At my suggestion, they finally ordered a conservative fluid bolus and electrolyte repletion. Despite the bolus, her blood pressure continued in the low 80s, and her heart rate was touching the 30s with more frequent premature ventricular contractions (PVCs). Again, I voiced my concerns with no change to the current plan. I reached out to the nursing supervisor who, upon hearing Mrs. Montgomery's story, became concerned and called the rapid response team and the medical senior to provide support and re-evaluate the patient's condition.

I reviewed Mrs. Montgomery's clinical profile and my observations in detail with the nursing supervisor and medical senior, and they agreed with my assessment. The vascular team returned to the bedside upset that I had reached out to another service and refused to consider transferring Mrs. Montgomery. They were very concerned the surgical attending would be upset that his post-op patient had to be transferred to an ICU. As the medical and surgical teams discussed Mrs. Montgomery's plan, I continued monitoring her as her blood pressure continued down to the 70s. I reminded them of Mrs. Montgomery's clinical profile and the need for ICU monitoring to meet her deteriorating status.

Eventually, the surgical team agreed, and Mrs. Montgomery was transferred to the SICU, where she was fluid resuscitated and stabilized over the next 2 days. I believe my ability to recognize a trend and my confidence in initiating a thorough assessment and anticipating problems helped ensure Mrs. Montgomery's health and healing.

When I was a new nurse, I thought understanding theory and being compassionate were the keys to good care. It was very intimidating not to agree with a surgeon, or team of surgeons, until I realized the value of my own expertise. In those moments of medical crisis when families aren't able to be at the bedside and patients aren't able to speak for themselves, I am the expert, and my voice is their voice. I had to find the confidence in my own clinical skills and knowledge to do what I knew was best for my patient—to be reminded of the person beyond the patient. When tension is high and decisions are being made quickly, sometimes making your voice heard when no one is listening can seem like the most daunting thing to do. But it might also be the thing your patient needs the most.

Commentary

This narrative shows how experienced clinicians' past experience informs their practice. Theodora recognized a pattern that told her that although Mrs. Montgomery might have momentarily stabilized, she was at risk for decompensating. While her well-respected and knowledgeable colleagues referred to Mrs. Montgomery's past baseline and current state, Theodora remained unconvinced. This narrative reflects a common issue that clinicians face as they advocate for a patient. Theodora managed the conflict by focusing on her assessment, available data, the patient's condition, and calling in resources for consultation. She was comfortable in managing the conflict.

Reflective Questions

- In many ways, the surgical team did not see the same patient as Theodora did. How do you try to get others to see the patient as you do? What do you think gets in the way of that happening?

- Theodora felt that she was not being heard and her concerns were being minimized. How do you react to these uncomfortable situations?

- After an emotional event like this, where talented smart people disagree on the management of a patient, would you speak to members of the team to debrief?

- What do you think can be done to create opportunities for nurses, physicians, and other members of the team to learn how to collaborate in effective ways?

If You Wish It, It Just Might Happen

Meaghan Costello, PT   **Practice level: Advanced Clinician**
Physical Therapist

Dennis was a 14-year-old boy with cystic fibrosis (CF) admitted from his doctor's office with complaints of worsening cough, shortness of breath (SOB), and fevers for 2 weeks. Dennis's mom, a single parent, had older twin boys who also have CF. I met Dennis on the day of his admission and was consulted to evaluate and assist with airway clearance. I had treated many adults and children with CF; however, this admission would present a significant challenge for the family and healthcare providers involved.

During my chart review, I became alarmed at the decrease in Dennis's pulmonary function tests (PFTs) since they had been taken 6 months prior. Dennis had also lost a significant amount of weight and hadn't grown in height. Notes in his medical record showed that doctors, social workers, nurses, and dieticians all shared concerns about Dennis's health and the number of doctor's visits that had been cancelled. For this reason, a claim of medical neglect was filed with the Department of Social Services (DSS). Dennis's mom was aware that DSS was notified, and the medical team and social worker stressed that this was to get Dennis's mom some help, as she had three very sick boys. I recognized that the claim could affect the trust Dennis and his mom had in the team caring for him.

I introduced myself to Dennis and his mom. Dennis was sitting in bed, watching TV and texting. Dennis immediately told me he couldn't do physical therapy (PT); he was too tired and had stomach pains. I noticed he didn't make any eye contact with me. I asked Dennis what his normal regimen was for airway clearance. He simply stated, "Chest PT." Dennis's mom elaborated that someone usually came to the house, but the boys weren't always there. As the conversation progressed, I gathered more information and gained insight into Dennis's mom's beliefs. She said that Dennis was sick; he wouldn't have quantity of life, but she wanted him to have quality of life and not feel that he was sick. She said that if Dennis turned his tube feed off at night so he didn't feel full in the morning, she couldn't make him turn it on. She couldn't make him take his medications after she reminded him, and he started to become defensive. I explained that my role was to help Dennis be able to do the things he loved without becoming so short of breath and help him feel better.

At this point, Dennis and his mom agreed to let me evaluate him, and I discovered multiple cardiovascular and musculoskeletal impairments. Dennis presented with abnormal lung sounds and increased resting respiratory rate with low oxygen saturations. He had impaired posture and poor muscle strength. Due to his nutritional status, he had very poor muscle definition, and I knew from reading the literature that patients with CF can also develop osteopenia. As part of my evaluation, I asked Dennis what his goals were. He looked at me and asked if I was serious. When he realized I was, he said to be on the freshman baseball team. I said that if we worked as a team, that could be one of our goals, but he didn't appear to believe me.

Dennis would be at our hospital for at least 2 weeks of IV antibiotics to address the infection in his lungs. Due to the severity of his impairments, I set up a plan of care that included PT twice a day for airway clearance and aerobic conditioning as soon as Dennis could tolerate it. Aerobic conditioning is an excellent mode of airway clearance, and I anticipated that Dennis's aerobic capacity was impaired. I discussed the plan of care that included his goal of being on the baseball team with Dennis and his mom, and they were in agreement.

Dennis presented a very tough exterior, but throughout the course of our treatments, he was able to trust me and open up a lot. I learned that although he was the youngest, he took on a great deal of responsibility for the family and worried a lot about being a burden to his mom. I also had many conversations with Dennis's mom regarding education about the importance of airway clearance, nutritional support, and aerobic conditioning. Dennis's mom continued to state that she didn't want to do interventions that would make Dennis feel that he was sick—she wanted to focus on his quality of life. She couldn't reconcile how these interventions would keep Dennis healthy and out of the hospital, thereby improving his quality of life. I recognized she couldn't set healthy expectation for Dennis, so I focused on Dennis and playing baseball.

There are many methods for airway clearance, and Dennis was familiar with percussion and vibration. He reported that he didn't like that method, and his perception was that it didn't help. The literature supports numerous methods, but the "best" one is the one the patient will actually do. I explained to Dennis the different options and allowed him to process the information and ask questions. He was willing to try various methods, and our active experimentation began. Dennis tried nebulizers, postural drainage, different breathing techniques, and an Acapella (an airway clearance device). He found fault with all of them. Taking his feedback into account, I decided to combine two methods, active-cycle breathing, which had left him lightheaded, and the Acapella, which would slow his breathing down. This was quite effective; he had no complaints and was willing to try it. I knew this was time well invested to find a method that Dennis could and would use. I knew if he was involved in making the decision, he'd be adherent.

After his third day in the hospital, Dennis was gaining weight nicely. I was concerned about his strength and anticipated aerobic-capacity impairments. I spoke with the dietician about his calories and weight gain. We developed a plan that if he stayed the same or lost weight, we'd cut back on his exercise. But if he continued to make gains, we would continue my exercise prescription.

I wasn't sure how much Dennis would be able to exercise, so I performed a modified Bruce protocol to assess his aerobic capacity. I explained that we'd do this again as he neared discharge to measure his progress. Dennis was only able to exercise for 6 minutes due to dyspnea on exertion (DOE) and a heart rate of 85% of max. I calculated Dennis's target heart rate for aerobic conditioning, which he would reach with moderately paced walking. After exercise, he mobilized a lot of secretions. Dennis made gains, adding incline to the treadmill and increasing his speed. During his aerobic conditioning, I measured his hemodynamic response, including heart rate, blood pressure, respiratory rate, oxygen saturation, and his perception of DOE and rate of perceived exertion (RPE). I started teaching Dennis how to use these scales appropriately so he could independently guide his exercise level post-discharge.

I prescribed an exercise program to improve his posture as he was forward flexed with rounded shoulders, which can impact the ventilatory system. Dennis had strength impairments, so we devised a strength-training program. We started using dumbbells in front of a mirror so he could see his posture. This was a great way for Dennis to receive feedback. He was making excellent gains in aerobic conditioning via treadmill walking, so I suggested he start jogging. He initially said it was impossible. I related his training to baseball and his ability to run the bases or field the ball. He was willing to try and managed to run for 2 minutes. I continually gave Dennis positive feedback, and slowly he began to develop self-confidence. I was so proud when he started being able to jog for 15 to 20 minutes.

During these sessions, Dennis would ask me a lot of questions, not just about exercise, but about CF. He again said he didn't want to worry his mom, and he thought his stomach started to hurt when he worried about that. He had been evaluated for this, and the team felt it was stress-related, though his mother didn't agree. I saw that Dennis trusted me. I shared with him that exercise helped control my stress. Sure enough, as his exercise increased, his complaints of stomach pain decreased.

Dennis was starting to take responsibility for his own health by the end of the 2 weeks, even after hearing the disappointing news that his hospitalization was being prolonged for continued care. During one of my visits, Dennis had about five friends visiting in his room. When most teenagers have visitors, they don't want to participate in physical therapy. I gave him the option of exercising later. I suggested he could do something other than running, or his friends could come with us. But he turned to his friends and said, "Sorry, I have to exercise."

I asked Dennis what his goals were besides playing baseball. He was initially confused, but when I said he should have goals for himself in addition to playing baseball, he said he wanted to be able to run for 30 minutes. And on day 14 he met that goal!

Dennis told me he really enjoyed running, and I encouraged him to keep at it. I told him the CF Foundation has a running scholarship for college. Every 7 days I re-evaluated Dennis's impairments, and he made excellent gains in posture, strength, pulmonary/ventilator status, and aerobic conditioning. I stressed the importance of continuing his exercise at home and asked how he intended to track his progress. Dennis wanted to use a calendar system. We set up a monthly calendar, and on each day we entered which exercise he'd do that day. I included pages for him to track distance run, heart rate, DOE, his strength program, and stretches. Dennis loved Chuck Norris, so I found a picture of him exercising and put it on the cover of his binder.

Dennis was discharged on day 16, with DSS follow-up. I was worried that once home, he might fall back into his old habits. I gave him the name of one of our outpatient therapists, who sees patients at the CF clinic to further reinforce carry-over at home.

I ran into Dennis one day in the main corridor as he was going to a doctor appointment with his mom. He was very excited that he'd made the summer baseball team, was playing, and felt great. He promised that he was using the Acapella every day, and he was still using the binder to keep track of his exercise program. And I'm happy to report that he's training to run a 3-mile road race in his hometown.

Commentary

When Meaghan first meets Dennis, he was immersed in his video game, responding in brief statements—a typical teenager. Yet his mother's love and anxiety that he will soon die was preventing him from being a teenager. Meaghan recognizes that her focus could not be on convincing his mom; rather, it needed to be on partnering with Dennis to push himself and to dream of being on the baseball team.

To move from dream to reality takes all of Meaghan's skill, past experience, and clinical knowledge to create a treatment plan that Dennis would adhere to, particularly in the face of his mother's ambivalence. Meaghan built on interventions that worked for Dennis in the past; she developed creative solutions by mixing and matching treatments that would move Dennis to managing CF independently.

Reflective Questions

- How do you instill hope in a patient that his quality of life could improve?

- Meaghan was extremely creative in developing a treatment plan for Dennis—one that he would adhere to. Can you describe the outcome of cases where you have mixed and matched treatments to suit the patient's needs?

- Have you had to balance developing a treatment plan that might not be the most effective, but is one that the patient could adhere to?

Creating Space for Hope

Stephen Joyce, RN   **Practice level: Advanced Clinician**
Clinical Nurse, Surgical Intensive Care

On a beautiful, late-summer day, Mr. Carson, a 21-year-old, experienced skydiver jumped out of a plane using a new experimental parachute. Halfway through the jump, the chute folded in on itself, and Mr. Carson hit the ground going approximately 60 miles an hour.

I was the resource nurse when Mr. Carson was admitted to the Surgical Intensive Care Unit. He was diagnosed with a subdural and probable diffuse axonal injury. Surprisingly, he had an intact spinal cord with only a fracture of T-12, which didn't require any surgical intervention, and extensive skull and facial fractures. He was ventilated with multiple lines and an intracranial bolt to monitor his intracranial pressure (ICP).

As I assisted in admitting Mr. Carson, the ophthalmologist entered the room, asking to dilate Mr. Carson's pupils. I told him that at this point, Mr. Carson required close monitoring of his neuro exam and that dilating his pupils would prevent us from doing that; I asked him to speak with the neurosurgical resident regarding the timing of the dilation. One role nurses play is coordinator of the many services required to care for patients—nurses see the whole patient. After discussion with the neurosurgical resident, the decision was made to dilate Mr. Carson's eyes because he had the bolt in place. Leaving work that night, I asked the resource nurse to assign me to care for Mr. Carson the next day.

The next day I found that Mr. Carson's mom, who lived out of state, had arrived along with his sister. They were very worried about him and his prognosis. I told them I'd schedule a meeting with all members of the team to discuss Mr. Carson's care and treatment. I also told them I'd ask the social worker to meet with them as they dealt with this trauma. Mr. Carson's family was calmer after our discussion, and I encouraged them to go to the cafeteria for breakfast, which they agreed to do. I've found that taking the time to develop a trusting relationship with families allows them to relax and care for themselves—they know you'll be there to take care of their family member.

Mr. Carson's neurological status had not changed overnight, and the risk that he'd develop a subdural hematoma remained high. He would require daily CT scans and hourly monitoring of his neuro status and ICP. I saw the neurosurgery team across the unit and turned off Mr. Carson's Propofol in anticipation of their arrival. He was on a high dose of Propofol, an anesthetic agent, which can take up to 20 minutes to clear. So, if the team is in a rush, the medication can affect the accuracy of the exam. At the appropriate time, I called the residents from the ICU and trauma team into Mr. Carson's room. I've found that interpretation of neuro exams can vary greatly. One person will call withdrawal purposeful; the other might not. It's better to get everyone in the room so there's a common understanding and visualization of the exam. Off the Propofol, Mr. Carson had purposeful movements only with his left arm.

Mr. Carson's pupils concerned me in that they remained dilated a whole day after the ophthalmologist had dilated them. His ICP remained good—in fact, too good; at times he was in negative numbers and had a good tracing. The team was fine with his numbers because they weren't high. I wasn't fine with the numbers. It is one thing to get a negative number when the patient is awake and participating in the neuro exam; it's another to get a negative number on a patient like Mr. Carson, who cannot participate in the exam, and you're worried about herniation. I continued to push, and the neurosurgeon finally agreed and switched the fiberoptic cable; cables can sometimes migrate and give an inaccurate reading.

The cause of Mr. Carson's injury and his neuro exam raised many questions for his family and the team about what Mr. Carson's quality of life would be if he survived. I told the family we wouldn't have a clear picture of who Mr. Carson would be for at least 6 to 12 months. But I had hope.

Hope came from having watched a 20-year-old woman walk into the unit 7 months after suffering a similar injury. At that time, the team had discussed withdrawing care; then, 7 months later, she was standing in the unit thanking us. She had returned to school, had a slight limp, and some short-term memory loss, but she was living her life. And there have been other people who've beaten the odds.

I knew I had to keep the family's hopes alive during these tough first few weeks, so I consulted a physician from Physical Medicine who had treated many young patients. Although it might have been early to involve him, I knew what his knowledge, experience, and, most importantly, his compassion would mean for this family.

I reviewed the case with him, and after examining Mr. Carson, he met with the family. He reinforced the need for time but was also able to prognosticate what Mr. Carson would be like and what he would need as he recovered. I saw the family relax as this talented and experienced physician met with them regularly.

Slowly, Mr. Carson stabilized, the bolt and the ventilator were removed, and plans were made for discharge to a general care neurology unit. I had hoped Mr. Carson would show more improvement in his neurological exam; he continued to move only his arm with purposeful movement. I know he still has a ways to go in his healing, and I look forward to hearing about his progress.

Commentary

In this narrative Steve demonstrated nurses' critical role as integrators, navigators, coordinators, communicators, advocates, and care providers. He looked beyond the specific intervention—say, the dilation of Mr. Carson's pupils—to how this intervention would impact the monitoring of his labile neurological status. His concern for ICP numbers that were "too good" demonstrated that he was not fooled by what the monitor said; instead, he integrated those numbers with what the patient was experiencing. His advocacy and tenacity in addressing this issue allowed for a change in the plan and better care. Throughout this rapidly changing situation, Steve never forgot that Mr. Carson is part of a family who needed attention, comfort, and knowledge as they navigated this new world they and Mr. Carson had entered.

Reflective Questions

- When a patient or family asks what the future holds, it can be challenging to know what to say and how much to say. Can you think of a similar situation you have experienced? What did you say? How did you know what to say?

- Do you react solely to the measurements that various medical devices provide, or do you assess the patient's current situation as well? What are the dangers in relying on "the numbers"?

- In some situations, it's critical for clinicians to "continue to push." What do you do and say in such situations? What do you do if the team does not respond?

Creating a New Normal

Brenda Pignone, RN   **Practice level: Clinical Scholar**
Clinical Nurse, General Surgery

When I decided to accept a position on a surgical/trauma unit 18 years ago, I knew I'd be caring for patients facing serious, life-changing situations. Many are able to return to "normal lives." Others, such as Ms. Abbott, suffer such severe trauma that their day-to-day lives will be anything but normal.

Ms. Abbott was a 50-year-old woman who'd been in a high-speed motor-vehicle accident while driving in another state. She suffered severe spinal-cord injury, traumatic brain injury, small subdural hematoma, and a fracture of a finger on her right hand. She was stabilized at a nearby hospital and then transferred to the Surgical ICU at MGH. Two days after being admitted, she was taken to surgery for a T-1 laminectomy and open reduction of her spinal fracture. Ms. Abbott was paraplegic and would be required to wear a spinal brace for up to 12 weeks. She was transferred to a general surgical unit when her condition stabilized. Her finger had been splinted, and her subdural hematoma was resolving. On her second day on the unit, she had an emergency tracheostomy and placement of a feeding tube secondary to her spinal-cord injury.

I began caring for Ms. Abbott the day after her tracheostomy. I knew, after reading her nursing assessment and plan of care, that she was going to need an experienced nurse. In report, I learned that Ms. Abbott had had a difficult night with nightmares about the accident. She required a great deal of emotional support and physical care due to her injuries. Upon entering her room, I went to the head of the bed and leaned over so she could make eye contact with me. I immediately saw the fear and anxiety in her eyes. I introduced myself and told her I'd be her nurse for the next 12 hours. After traumatic brain injury, many patients need constant reminders of the plan of care. I assessed her physical needs. Her vital signs were stable; her lungs sounded clear; her trach was secure; her position was comfortable; her brace was properly fitted; IV lines, feeding tube, and Foley catheter were checked, secured, and dated; her Morse Fall Scale and Braden Scores were recorded; and her pain was under control. I was able to make these assessments while continuing to provide emotional support to Ms. Abbott.

After meeting with the surgical team during morning rounds, I spent time with Ms. Abbott and her husband discussing Ms. Abbott's physical and emotional issues and helping staff manage the situation. Both Ms. Abbott and her husband spoke about how important it was for her to be able to touch her surroundings and her caregivers—it helped remind her of where she was and reassured her she was safe. Ms. Abbott shared that because she could no longer feel her legs, her sense of touch was vital to her sense of "who she was at that moment."

Ms. Abbott was a professional French horn player. She needed to feel she could still use her arms, so she'd constantly move her arms seeking things to touch. I quickly arranged a meeting with Ms. Abbott, her husband, the nurse practitioner, the social worker, and the psychiatric clinical nurse specialist. With this new information, I felt it was important for Ms. Abbott to have a sitter who could sit by her bed at night. When Ms. Abbott reached out, the sitter could remind her that she was at the hospital, that she'd been in an accident, give her the date and time, and assure her that she was safe.

My colleagues and nursing director supported the plan, and it was a tremendous help to Ms. Abbott. Over the next few nights, her anxiety diminished, she felt more comfortable having a sitter, and she was able to sleep better during the night. Her need to use the call bell decreased as she developed trust with the sitters, knowing they would call a nurse if necessary. And with hourly rounds, both the patient and the sitter knew that someone would check in on her on a regular basis.

Ms. Abbott spent many weeks on our unit recovering from her spinal-cord injury. Because of the complexity of her care, I spent a great deal of time with her performing skin care, maintaining adequate pain relief, helping her learn to eat again, and performing chest physical therapy and respiratory toilet. After a few weeks, Ms. Abbott was able to come out of the brace and transfer to a wheelchair that she soon learned to roll by herself.

I helped initiate many consults for Ms. Abbott, including Psychiatry to help with her anxiety and post-traumatic stress syndrome; Pain Management to be sure that she was appropriately weaned from narcotics; and Physical and Occupational Therapy, Social Service, and Case Management so that she could transition smoothly into rehabilitation with no change in her plan of care.

Ms. Abbott had an incredible family that was very supportive. She was married with three children. One daughter was a senior in college and extremely supportive. She called every day and spent evenings with her mother at the hospital. Mr. Abbott and I discussed how important it was for Ms. Abbott's friends to visit. Visitors helped her relax. We created a list of visitors so I could remind Ms. Abbott who would be visiting her and for how long. I encouraged the evening staff (with Ms. Abbott's permission) to involve the daughter in her mom's care and show her what she would need to know to help care for her mom at home. Both Ms. Abbott and her daughter found this beneficial as we talked about what Ms. Abbott's "new normal" was going to be. Her daughter told me that after graduating, her goal was to design a new spinal brace that was simpler to use and more comfortable for patients.

The day Ms. Abbott was transferred to a rehabilitation facility, I spoke at length to the rehab nurse about the plan we had put in place to help Ms. Abbott with her anxiety. I was fortunate to be able to visit her at her rehab and see that she was progressing well.

Ms. Abbott inspired me with her courage and strength. I care for trauma patients every day, and I always incorporate my experience and expertise in critical-incident stress management into my care. I knew it was important for Ms. Abbott to understand how trauma affects the body, both physically and emotionally. Trauma releases chemicals that increase anxiety, distort our ability to make decisions, and create fear. I try to help trauma patients minimize the effects of stress by encouraging them to sleep, maintain proper nutrition, surround themselves with family and friends, and seek professional help when needed. I assured Ms. Abbott—as I do all my patients—that these reactions are normal responses to stress. Validating these responses is vital to the emotional and physical well-being of patients long after their hospital stay is over.

Commentary

How do you rebuild a life? Slowly, and with a lot of guidance, support, and understanding. Brenda's expert knowledge and interventions allowed Ms. Abbott and her family to be able to imagine and plan for the next chapter of their lives. It would have been easy to focus on Ms. Abbott's extensive physical injuries, but Brenda gave equal attention to her mental and emotional needs. As Brenda pointed out, trauma triggers a number of responses, and she skillfully and with great compassion guided them to this new life.

Reflective Questions

- In this narrative, Ms. Abbott said that touching was "vital to her sense of who she was at that moment." What does this statement tell you about her and where she was in her recovery?

- Brenda was very aware of not only where Ms. Abbott was in the moment but the trajectory of her recovery and future needs. How do you anticipate what those needs will be, even when the patient and family may be challenged to think that far ahead?

- Brenda developed an extensive plan to address Ms. Abbott's physical and emotional needs. How do you achieve buy-in from your colleagues to follow such a plan when you are not working?

- It is not only Ms. Abbott's life that was changed by this accident; it is also her family's and friends' lives. How do you support patients and their families both in the short term and the future?

In Eight Hours, a Life Is Changed

Katherine Fillo, RN   **Practice level: Clinical Scholar**
Clinical Nurse, General Medicine

The five units that make up the House Medicine Service are unique in that the patients on this service usually present with complex social, emotional, and physical needs. They often don't have access to primary care, so they end up using the emergency department (ED) for their healthcare needs, which are often acute and could have been prevented or managed with more timely intervention.

One patient, Mr. Flores, is a perfect example. Mr. Flores worked full time unloading trucks, but he wasn't eligible for health insurance due to his immigration status. While he had noticed increasing thirst, urination, and fatigue, he didn't seek care until he was brought into the ED by ambulance after losing consciousness.

I met Mr. Flores on the third day of admission. When I walked into his room at 7:30 a.m., he was already up, sitting in the chair, staring out the window. He greeted me hesitantly in English, and when I answered him in Spanish, a wave of relief spilled over his face. He had been admitted to general medical unit for diabetic ketoacidosis, and now, a little more than 48 hours later, it was determined that Mr. Flores would require insulin to manage his diabetes after discharge. He was likely to be discharged later that day. From reading the progress notes and the handoff from the nurse who cared for him the night before, I knew that Mr. Flores had many skills to learn in a short period of time. To help him learn, I needed to establish a therapeutic relationship; I needed to find out what was important to him.

As I performed my morning assessment, I asked Mr. Flores about his family and his work. He lived in a rooming house, and his only family in the United States was his younger sister, whom he adored; she lived down the street from him. He worried that he'd missed so much work he wouldn't be paid. I listened as he spoke. I asked Mr. Flores what he knew about diabetes, and in Spanish he replied, "Diabetes killed my mother." This statement was powerful and shed light on his understanding of the disease. Most of Mr. Flores's knowledge had come from watching his mother in El Salvador. He could tell me that diabetes had something to do with sugar, but not much more.

Mr. Flores reported that since coming to the hospital, he "felt normal." I explained that insulin had helped make him feel more energetic. I used the teach-back technique, having patients use their own words to explain a concept to ensure that they comprehend important information, and Mr. Flores was able to verbalize his understanding of the connection between insulin and his energy level.

I coached Mr. Flores in the use of the glucometer to check his blood sugar, and soon he successfully pricked his finger and placed a drop of blood onto the reader strip. This was evidence to me that he learned best when given small amounts of information at a time. I explained to Mr. Flores that he'd need to use a similar device at home to check his blood sugar every morning. He asked how much it would cost, and I realized that his lack of insurance would mean he'd have to pay for his medication and equipment himself.

The plan was for Mr. Flores to be discharged that afternoon, which meant I had less than 8 hours to advocate for Mr. Flores to receive follow-up services at a clinic near his home. I knew the clinic had bilingual staff and a dedicated diabetes program.

The junior resident and I discussed Mr. Flores's insulin regimen; I knew it would be important for Mr. Flores to be able to inject himself using the supplies he'd have available at home. I paged the endocrinologist who'd be making the final decision, and we had a conversation about Mr. Flores's latest blood sugars and discharge plan. I explained Mr. Flores's concern about the cost of the glucometer, and she offered to have a sample glucometer brought to the unit. I was excited that we had overcome one hurdle and were that much closer to a safe discharge plan. The junior resident wrote prescriptions for twice daily 70/30 insulin, syringes, testing strips, and lancets. I checked with our unit case manager to see if I could obtain a delayed payment voucher for the prescriptions, and she was happy to provide it.

I returned to Mr. Flores's room. I explained the plan, and Mr. Flores said that he was motivated to take care of himself and having "the machine" would help.

I asked how he'd be getting home, and he said his sister would be picking him up. I asked if she might like to learn how to give insulin injections, too, and Mr. Flores was receptive to the idea. I called his sister and planned for her to come in for a teaching session.

By noon, Mr. Flores's new glucometer had arrived. He was quickly able to demonstrate that he could check his blood sugar with minimal coaching. Because his glucose level was over 200, I got a bottle of insulin so he could practice drawing up the medication himself. Again, I used the teach-back/show-back method to walk him through the process of drawing up insulin and injecting himself. After a moment of apprehension, Mr. Flores successfully injected the needle into his abdomen.

Mr. Flores's sister arrived later that afternoon. I had printed out some materials on insulin injection and special diets for diabetics. Mr. Flores's sister was a petite and outgoing woman; she was eager to learn how to help him, and we quickly established a comfortable rapport. I was surprised at how much more lively Mr. Flores was with his sister present. She seemed to bring out his true character.

I encouraged Mr. Flores to show his sister what he'd learned about the glucometer and blood-sugar monitoring. This enabled me to gauge what Mr. Flores had retained from earlier in the day. I beamed with pride as I watched Mr. Flores show his sister how to prick his finger for a blood sample and then allowed her to do the same. When the glucometer read 145, Mr. Flores was able to interpret the results. "It's okay, not too much sugar."

I had them both practice drawing up the evening dose of insulin from the bottle I'd obtained earlier. Satisfied that both Mr. Flores and his sister were competent, I transitioned to teaching injection technique. They engaged in some classic sibling horseplay, with the sister pretending to be excited about injecting him with the needle. But when the moment arrived, Mr. Flores's sister was completely focused and took the task very seriously. She performed the task perfectly.

Mr. Flores and his sister left the hospital a half hour later. They were both grateful for the time I'd spent with them, and I was thrilled at their willingness to learn. I'm confident Mr. Flores returned home and to work without any complications. I know I met Mr. Flores and his family's needs to the best of my abilities. And most importantly, I'll incorporate the lessons I learned from Mr. Flores about involving family in discharge-teaching into my care of future patients.

Commentary

Kate needed to convey a great deal of information in a very short time in order to ensure Mr. Flores was discharged safely. And she expertly managed it all with Mr. Flores's well-being as her primary focus. She collaborated and directed other members of the team to ensure continuity; she used the evidence-based, teach-back technique to ensure Mr. Flores knew how to use the glucometer and self-administer insulin. She built on his close relationship with his sister to make sure he had the support he needed. And she did all this with compassion, with empathy, and as efficiently as possible.

Reflective Questions

- Mr. Flores has suffered with the symptoms of diabetes, lacks health coverage, and is worried about work. What issues and possible solutions would you have in the moment and in the future for Mr. Flores to maintain his health?

- In this narrative, Mr. Flores was successfully able to demonstrate the techniques he learned. What would you do if your patient was not able to successfully teach back and show back all that you had taught him?

- Mr. Flores had a willing and capable sister. Have you been in situations where family is unavailable or unwilling to participate in the care of their family member? If so, what do you do?

Summary

In this chapter, clinicians from across the disciplines shared with us their clinical knowledge and decision-making. We saw in these narratives how past experience informs their thinking and actions. For those clinicians new to the practice, recognition of what is occurring and how to effectively intervene requires greater analysis and guidance from more experience clinicians. Narratives from clinicians with more experience show a greater understanding of the whole situation, why it is occurring, and what needs to be done. There is great opportunity at these levels for the clinicians to reflect on "what they saw" and their decision-making. These conversations on their narrative allow for greater reflection, identification of further learning opportunities, and the sharing of experiential knowledge with others.

References

Benner, P. (1984). *From novice to expert: Excellence and power in clinical nursing practice.* Menlo Park, CA: Addison-Wesley.

Dreyfus, H. L., & Dreyfus, S. E., with Athanasiou, T. (1986). *Mind over machine.* New York, NY: Free Press.

Chapter 4

Theme of Practice: Teamwork and Collaboration

Through the development of effective relationships with unit-based colleagues and other members of the healthcare team, the best possible outcome is achieved for the patient and family.

IN THIS CHAPTER

- Stopping a moving train
- Listening even when it is hard to hear
- Setting the stage for effective learning
- Rallying support
- Laughing through the rough patches

The Importance of Teamwork and Collaboration

For many years, teamwork and collaboration addressed creating a positive work environment. Over the past decade, the role of teamwork and collaboration in quality and safety has brought new prominence (IOM, 2000, 2001, 2004; JCAHO, 2008) to the importance of a healthy environment of care. The narratives that clinicians at Massachusetts General Hospital (MGH) have written reflect how teamwork and collaboration are not only a critical theme in their personal development, but also how each clinician develops in his or her own comfort and approach to being part of a team.

Narratives—Entry Level of Practice

In their academic preparation, advanced beginners or Entry-level clinicians learn the value of teamwork and collaboration; yet, as they enter into practice, they often feel ill-prepared. Becoming a member of the team requires them to recognize and understand the various roles of the team members and to gain the confidence and credibility necessary to collaborate. Narratives at this stage often reflect the clinician's challenge of trying to fit in with the team. In unbundling the narratives, colleagues and leadership are able to dialogue with the clinician about each team member's role and how they can assist the novice clinician in addressing patient needs.

Narratives—Clinician Level of Practice

At the competent or Clinician level, the clinicians' narratives reflect their comfort in becoming part of the team and participating in interdisciplinary forums. Their narratives reflect the value they have for the team and openness to addressing issues and concerns with members of the team, though often they require the backup of others. In these narratives, it is possible to help the clinicians identify opportunities to further understand their role and work with other members of the team in accomplishing patient, professional, and organizational goals.

Narratives—Advanced Clinician Level of Practice

Narratives at the proficient or Advanced Clinician levels reflect a clinician who is known by other members of the team as someone who is knowledgeable and skilled, who seeks out opportunities to collaborate, and who is increasingly comfortable managing conflict. The ability to manage conflict at this level and the expert (Clinical Scholar) level reflects commitment to creating a healthy work environment in which all members are heard and respected—even when in disagreement.

Narratives—Clinical Scholar Level of Practice

Clinicians' narratives at the expert or Clinical Scholar levels reflect their confidence and authority in working with patients, families, and all members of the team. Their narratives reflect their generosity to elevating the practice of the entire team by teaching and with consultation. Their comfort with their own practice—with what they know and what they do not know—allows them to seek out consultation from others. They recognize that the true measure of collaboration is not when everyone agrees, but what occurs when they do not. Do they pull away or apart, or do they stay committed to doing what is in the best interest of the patient? Their narratives are rich in lessons on how clinicians can stay committed to the core value of patient-centeredness.

The narratives that follow describe the teamwork and collaboration theme of practice across the six disciplines and across the four levels of expertise, as described in Chapter 1. The unbundling through reflective questions, which follows a brief commentary on the narrative, allows you to reflect on your own practice or that of a colleague.

When the Patient Says It's Time

Lauren Aloisio, RN   **Practice level: Clinician**
Clinical Nurse, Medical/Surgical

Nursing has been described as "God's work," where life-and-death decisions are not out of the ordinary. There are certain moments in every nurse's career that become seared in his or her memory. I didn't comprehend the full meaning of those statements until I cared for Ms. Dilts. It was a major milestone in my nursing career, one I'll remember forever.

Ms. Dilts was a 46-year-old woman, wife, mother, friend, and avid church member. She came to the Cancer Center for chemotherapy and radiation therapy; she had a strong support system and discussed her condition openly and honestly with them. Her faith guided her throughout her treatment; her pastor and church community were consistently by her side.

Despite prolonged chemotherapy and radiation treatment, Ms. Dilts's cancer was aggressive and caused her significant pain. Her hospital admissions were becoming more frequent and longer in duration. Palliative Care employed exhaustive strategies to control her pain, but with little or no effect. Ironically, Ms. Dilts's pain was exacerbated by narcotics, so her options for pain relief were slim. End-of-life care was now a frequent topic of conversation. It was a subject Ms. Dilts didn't shy away from; she was brave and thorough in preparing her family and friends for her impending death. It was then, 6 months prior to her passing, that her doctors introduced the idea of palliative sedation.

The goal of palliative sedation is to bring an end to intractable pain, not hasten death. According to the *MGH Policy & Procedures Manual*, an intravenous sedative (such as Lorazepam, Midazolam, Propofol, or Pentobarbital) may be used to control intractable symptoms. Patients must have a "severe, chronic, life-threatening illness" in order for palliative sedation to be an option. The patient has control and makes the decision to begin the process.

During the discussion about palliative sedation, Ms. Dilts shared that when she slept, she felt no pain. But she was adamant that she would choose this option only as a last resort and that it would be her decision.

On our unit, caring for comfort-measures-only or end-of-life patients is not uncommon, but Ms. Dilts's care plan was different from what many of us were accustomed to. The night before I met her, Ms. Dilts had told her palliative care doctors that, "It was time." She made the informed decision to turn to palliative sedation to end her suffering, not her life. She wanted to see her closest family and friends prior to beginning the process the next day.

I began my 7:00 a.m. shift unaware of what my day would hold. The night resource nurse informed me that I was being assigned to Ms. Dilts for a reason. "I know you'll take extraordinary care of Ms. Dilts and her family," she said. "You'll be able to connect with them on the emotional level they'll need today."

Her words gave me a sense of pride and also a sense of duty to uphold my nursing practice. After receiving report, the lead doctor and social worker from Ms. Dilts's palliative care team approached me. They explained what palliative sedation was, talked about Ms. Dilts's complicated pain history, and described how the process would go. They stressed that they'd be available for any questions or issues I had. I felt a strong sense of support from them as well as from my nursing colleagues.

Throughout the day, I met with Ms. Dilts, her family, her pastor, and many other members of her inner circle. As I witnessed Ms. Dilts's intense suffering and inability to control her pain, I knew something had to be done. During the brief moments when she was able to sleep, Ms. Dilts did exhibit nonverbal indications that she was pain-free. It was clear in my nursing opinion that palliative sedation was the appropriate course of action for her situation. But if I'd had any doubts, the palliative care team was right there to answer my questions, help meet Ms. Dilts's needs, and engage in open dialogue.

Palliative sedation is not widely used. And although I had no prior experience with it, there wasn't a doubt in my mind that this was the best choice for Ms. Dilts.

During a large, emotionally charged family meeting, doctors described the palliative-sedation process and talked about what to expect. Fond memories of Ms. Dilts were shared, and a beautiful passage was read by her pastor. As I stood in the room filled with her closest family and friends, I felt such sorrow, but also an immense sense of responsibility. I would have the privilege of accompanying my ailing patient to a peaceful death. At the close of the meeting, all family members and members of the team were in agreement; they were emotionally ready to exchange their last words with Ms. Dilts.

Each loved one had an opportunity to say good-bye. It was truly an honor to be included in such an intimate and powerful part of Ms. Dilts's life. Though at times it felt intrusive, I knew her family looked to me as a kind of savior, as someone who was going to help bring an end to their loved one's suffering.

It took great strength to cross the threshold into Ms. Dilts's room. My own grandmother passed away 12 years ago, and there wasn't a moment that day that I didn't look to her for strength and guidance to help Ms. Dilts and her family.

After a time, I looked into the tear-filled eyes of my patient and her family and said, "It's time."

Ms. Dilts took a deep breath and looked at her husband and children, whom she adored. She squeezed their hands and said, "Remember, God is good; He is *so* good."

I asked if she was ready, and she nodded. I administered the drugs and began the drip at the prescribed dose; several titrations were necessary to keep her asleep. During each dose change, the palliative care team was by my side. Eventually, Ms. Dilts settled into a persistent, sedative, unconscious state. The palliative care team, my nursing colleagues, and I had provided a smooth, dignified process to end our patient's suffering.

Ms. Dilts lived approximately four more days after the initiation of palliative sedation. Her death was peaceful. The time Ms. Dilts spent preparing her loved ones for her passing helped a great deal in their ability to begin the grieving process.

I commend my nursing colleagues, the palliative care team, and nursing leadership for their incredible support in this effort. We helped a terminally ill patient find a peaceful, intentional escape from her intractable pain, something some say that only God can do.

Commentary

In this narrative Lauren articulates the moral and ethical decisions faced by clinicians every day. Lauren describes the thoughtful process Palliative Care and all members of the team went through as they raised the issue of palliative sedation with Ms. Dilts and her family. Ms. Dilts and her family were given the gift of time to consider this intervention and when she would know the time was right for this intervention.

Lauren did not view her role as merely administering medication; it is clear from this narrative she needed to understand and know Ms. Dilts and that her decision to undergo this intervention was informed and made on her own. Throughout the day, Lauren was an active participant and observer in the discussion and realized that Ms. Dilts was ready to be free from pain and was at peace with her decision. It is through that understanding that Lauren, with the support of the team, administered the medication with the goal to alleviate Ms. Dilts's suffering.

Reflective Questions

- Ms. Dilts, her family, and the team had been having the discussion on palliative for many months; Lauren entered into this conversation on the day it was to be implemented. What helps you to know that the plan decided upon is the "right" plan and that you could participate in it?

- Do you have any moral or ethical concerns about participating in starting palliative sedation? What resources can you call upon to help you address those concerns?

- Lauren wrote that comfort-measure-only patients were not uncommon on her unit. How might this situation differ from caring for other patients who are terminally ill and receiving sedation?

Always Be Prepared

Gloria Mendez-Carcamo, RRT   **Practice level: Clinician**
Respiratory Therapist

As a respiratory therapist, I've developed many collaborative relationships with nurses and physicians, so I'm often consulted for asthma instruction, educating patients on how to manage newly placed tracheostomies after they are discharged, and assisting with oxygen therapy. I'm frequently consulted by nurses and physicians to help assess and treat patients in respiratory distress and respiratory failure. When I respond to these calls, I'm confident in my ability to assess the patient and make recommendations to the team as to the most appropriate respiratory therapy interventions. I'll never forget one seemingly routine page that quickly turned into a close call.

I responded to the page by phone to inquire about the situation. I wanted to be able to anticipate any equipment I might need and consider potential treatment options. I was told I was needed right away to assess a patient in respiratory distress. I couldn't get any more details because the nurse who paged me was in the midst of tending to the patient at the bedside. I quickly stopped by the Respiratory Care office and grabbed a non-invasive ventilator in anticipation of acute congestive heart failure (CHF) or exacerbation of chronic obstructive pulmonary disease (COPD).

When I arrived on the unit, I was met by several nurses who directed me to the patient's room. As I approached the door, I heard a sound that immediately eliminated CHF or COPD exacerbation as the source of the problem. The stridor told me that this patient would likely need a more complex intervention. When I stepped into the room, I saw a 40-year-old man sitting in bed with both elbows perched on the bedside table (tripod position), gasping for air. There was panic in his eyes. The distinctive, high-pitched sound he was producing suggested severe acute upper-airway obstruction. This was a medical emergency.

The nurse told me he had developed difficulty breathing a few minutes after initiating his first chemotherapy session. The chemotherapy was terminated, but the patient continued to gasp for air. I knew the treatment for stridor was aerosolized epinephrine to minimize or slow the swelling of the airway. Epinephrine can provide rapid relief of subglottic edema and, in some cases, breathing rapidly improves. A physician had already asked the nurse to get epinephrine and a nebulizer, so it was there when I arrived. We immediately administered the treatment. But I suspected, because of the severity of the stridor, that it wasn't going to open his airway enough to relieve his respiratory distress. I asked the team to stat page the anesthesia team for probable intubation.

While waiting for the anesthesia team, we elevated the patient's head to 45 degrees for optimal airway position. I asked one of the nurses to call my supervisor and request a tank of helium-oxygen (heliox). The low-density mixture can improve breathing in the case of severe partial upper-airway obstruction. I started to make the necessary preparations for intubation, but the patient became increasingly restless. His stridor became more acute, to the point where he started grunting and gasping for air. The anesthesia team arrived and immediately started to intubate. But when the attending anesthesiologist assessed the airway, he saw that the throat was completely closed. He called for the surgical airway team, stat.

While we waited for the team to arrive, the anesthesiologist held a resuscitation mask in place while I manually ventilated the patient, which was extremely difficult due to the obstructed airway. The anesthesiologist had to kneel on the bed to achieve a tight enough mask seal while I forced air into the airway. As we worked, we saw the patient's chest rise and his oxygen saturation level improve. Within a few minutes, the surgical team arrived and prepared for an *emergent surgical cricothyrotomy*, a procedure where a tube is passed through the neck into the trachea.

The surgeon performed the procedure in less than 5 minutes. After the airway was established and the patient was ventilating better, his vital signs returned to normal. The emergency was over. Everybody in the room—surgeons, physicians, nurses, and respiratory therapists—breathed a sigh of relief (as did the patient!). I had worked closely with this surgeon before. After discussing the plan of care with the team, he turned to me and asked if I was satisfied with the tracheostomy. I told him everything looked fine; there didn't seem to be any issues with the airway.

"Then I can leave," he said. "I know the patient is in good hands."

I connected the patient to a transport ventilator, and we transferred the patient to the intensive care unit.

A few weeks later, I saw this patient again on the same unit where I had been paged to care for him. This time, it was a very different encounter. He recognized me and thanked me for caring for him in a very scary situation. He was now ready to try a speaking valve, and I was the respiratory therapist assigned to him. A *speaking valve* is a valve placed on the tracheostomy tube to assess a patient's ability to breathe in through the tube and out through his/her upper airway. Utilizing a speaking valve enables us to assess the patient's level of recovery from a prior upper-airway obstruction. I placed the speaking valve, and the patient was able to breathe comfortably and talk for the first time since his emergency tracheostomy procedure. The speech-language pathologist was consulted to assess his risk of aspiration. After assessing him together for a few days, we recommended removal of his tracheostomy tube. The tube was removed, and the patient was discharged 2 weeks later.

This case reinforced my belief that teamwork is essential in the care of the patient, and especially in emergent situations. It's much less stressful when clinicians from different disciplines work together seamlessly and effectively, as they certainly did in this case. And it's nice to be recognized and appreciated as part of the team that provides excellent, patient-focused care.

Commentary

From the moment Gloria received that "routine" page, she started anticipating what to expect and what she would need. Her intuition, experience, and preparation were pivotal to the outcomes of this patient. Because she and the other members of the team responded quickly and efficiently in this critical situation, there was no wasted time and no delayed action. Instinct and expert practice took over. Every time a clinician has the benefit of a skilled team at his or her side in an emergent situation, it builds confidence and readiness for the next time. Clearly, Gloria was an integral part of a very skilled team.

Reflective Questions

- You may know from the moment you see or hear a patient what is happening and what will be needed. Have you been in a similar situation in the past? If so, what did you learn from those experiences that allowed you to practice so effortlessly moving forward?

- In this narrative the team was challenged to get the best seal possible in order to successfully ventilate the patient with the mask. Can you describe how hands should be placed and the best method of bagging to make each breath effective?

- The surgeon asked Gloria if she was satisfied with the tracheostomy. What can go wrong with an emergency tracheostomy, and what might you look for to make sure everything is fine?

Not So Fast...

Rebecca Santos Inzana, SLP   **Practice level: Clinician**
Speech–Language Pathologist

This story begins when I received a consult from the neurology service asking me to assess communication and swallow function as well as answer a specific question: "Does the patient need a PEG?" *Percutaneous endoscopic gastrostomy* (PEG) is a procedure in which a tube (PEG tube) is passed into a patient's stomach through the abdominal wall, most commonly to provide a means of feeding when oral intake is not adequate.

The patient was Hope. At 87, Hope was widowed and lived independently at home, enjoyed going out to eat, singing, socializing with family and friends, and was well-known for her feisty-yet-lovable personality. Overall she was in decent health, with a history of hypertension and hyperlipidemia. She had a large and loving family, including her four children, their loving spouses, and her many grandchildren who lived nearby. Ironically, no one was with her when she stroked.

Hope was her usual vibrant self when she was last seen at 7:00 p.m. the night of her stroke. Her daughter, Nancy, called at 11:00 p.m., as she did every night, to wish Hope good night. This time there was no answer. Nancy arrived at her mother's home to find her slumped over in the chair, coughing on her own vomit and unable to speak. Nancy immediately called 911, and Hope was brought to the emergency department. Unfortunately, while it was clear Hope had suffered a stroke, she was not a candidate for tissue plasminogen activator (t-PA), which dissolves blood clots, because she was outside the time window, and the clot in her middle cerebral artery had already done the majority of damage it was going to do.

During neurology rounds the next day, I listened as the physician introduced Hope as a patient who had a big stroke, had aspiration pneumonia, and wasn't going to be able to swallow. The team needed to clarify with the family whether the patient would want a gastrostomy tube or transition to comfort care. I told the physician that I would be meeting and evaluating Hope that morning, and, without entirely refuting the concerns about her swallow, suggested that it appeared to be a bit premature to go down the PEG versus comfort-measures-only route just yet, as it hadn't been 48 hours and her exam could change. I told the team that I was encouraged for a functional swallow because, according to the nurse, Hope was managing her own secretions.

After rounds, I reviewed Hope's scans and, based on those scans, made several predictions on her recovery. She would have significant aphasia, which would prevent her from verbally communicating. I also predicted that she would have some level of motor and sensory deficits, though I believed it was possible that her swallowing mechanism was adequately preserved to be functional.

After checking in with her nurse, I entered the room and introduced myself to Hope and her four children. The children were appropriately anxious and immediately began to ask questions. I explained to Hope and her family that I was there to assess Hope's swallowing function in order to determine how long it might be before Hope would be able to eat. No sooner had I mentioned eating when her children described Hope's love of food, talking, and singing. They asked me if she would be able to return to doing all of her favorite things. I assured them that I would do everything to make that happen.

I turned my full attention to Hope, who was lying in bed, looking exhausted. She looked at me, and although she was unable to speak, her eyes were very communicative, acknowledging me but exuding fatigue as well as some fear. I took her hand and introduced myself, explaining my role and why I was seeing her. I paid special attention to my intonation and gestures in my own communication, as I was unsure at this point how much Hope could comprehend.

The first thing I noticed was how quickly and audibly Hope was breathing. I asked her family if this was her normal breathing; they said that while she did wheeze on exhalation with an occasional cough, her current pattern was very different. Her current breathing pattern concerned me because airway protection during swallowing is difficult to maintain during compromised ventilation. This was key information to factor into her overall plan.

Narrating my actions and intentions for Hope and her family, I began the exam. Hope was unable to speak, though she could occasionally make some sounds on command. Her voice was strong, and her cough was sharp. I observed that she spontaneously swallowed her saliva throughout our session, also an excellent prognostic indicator of preserved swallow function. As Hope was still breathing heavily, I elected to give her only one ice chip, just to see how she would orally manipulate it and how long it would take her to swallow. It was a calculated risk; I knew if she did aspirate it, the quantity would be benign and therefore a minimal threat to her pulmonary status. Hope opened her mouth willingly, took the ice chip, chewed it, and swallowed. She did get increasingly short of breath with this activity, however, and had a dry cough before and after this trial; I wondered if she was perhaps silently aspirating.

I explained to Hope's family that she had many positive factors that indicated a return to oral feedings, but that before I could progress her feedings, we needed to get her to breathe more comfortably. The family was grateful and more hopeful after my visit, and I told them I would continue to work with Hope.

I left the room and sought out the resident caring for Hope. Before I could share my findings, the physician said, "I am not sure how this is going to work because the family said she wouldn't want a gastrostomy tube." Recognizing this as a teaching opportunity that could impact the way the resident approached Hope and other patients in the future, I explained that the findings on Hope's scan as well as her current swallowing exam were encouraging that Hope would return to oral feeding. My concern, I explained, was Hope's respiratory status. I recommended a modified barium study to determine if Hope was aspirating.

The physician was amenable to this plan, which would also buy Hope a few more days from a neuro perspective to hopefully spontaneously recover more function so that we'd have the best chance at a successful exam on which we could base decisions on her management and rehabilitation.

The next day, I was paged by Hope's nurse that Hope had pulled out her NG tube and she needed my help in giving Hope her essential medications by mouth. Together Hope's nurse and I cleaned Hope's mouth and safely delivered the needed medication. Unfortunately, later that morning, Hope's respiratory status worsened. I immediately spoke with the resident and told her that we were going in the wrong direction. I told the resident that Hope was not exhibiting the signs of pneumonia and advocated for a chest X-ray to rule out other causes for her distress. After discussion, the physician ordered the chest X-ray and with it found an increase in Hope's pulmonary edema. She was diuresed, and by the next morning she was breathing comfortably, had stopped wheezing entirely, and was medically stable for me to work with. I found her alert, engaged, and swallowing her medication crushed in pudding. I performed a modified barium swallow that was consistent with her exam and stroke and a mild dysphagia.

Hope and her family were elated with the results and became even happier when Hope sang "Happy Birthday" (this is an automatic task that engages the right brain function to encourage verbal input). Needless to say, the family members were in tears to hear Hope sing.

The next day, Hope was ready for discharge. Surrounded by her family, she was alert, breathing comfortably, eating well on her special diet, communicating with gestures, and participating with the other therapies. The family knew there was still work to do to allow Hope to recover as fully as possible, but they are armed with knowledge, determination, and limitless love. I also know that Hope taught her physician a valuable lesson in not rushing to judgment.

Commentary

The changes in the healthcare system are putting pressure on clinicians to safely and efficiently manage patient "throughput." Recovery and recuperation occur at home or at a lower level of care. This narrative allows us to reflect on how we balance efficiency with allowing the patient to "declare themselves."

That was the situation Rebecca found herself in as she advocated for her patient and educated her physician colleague on the recovery of a patient with this particular type of stroke. She tempered the immediate response for a PEG and instead, after reviewing the scans and her exam of the patient, prognosticated on the patient's recovery and function.

Rebecca was clearly comfortable in this changing clinical situation and quickly recognized that Hope's respiratory problems were not aspiration but rather cardiac in nature, and her advocacy for additional imaging prevented continued antibiotic treatment as well as initiated a swallowing study that allowed Hope to eat.

Rebecca's relentless focus on maximizing Hope's recovery is evident throughout this narrative, but perhaps no more so than when Rebecca was engaged with Hope and her family. Rebecca took time to learn who Hope is. Her curiosity about Hope opened up an opportunity to learn about foods Hope loves, social supports, and her personality. All that information enriches the story of who Hope is and gives hope for her recovery.

Reflective Questions

- Patients' families frequently ask clinicians to prognosticate on the patient's recovery, which can be difficult as you balance hope, reality, and the unknown. How do you know what to say and how to say it?

- How can you learn to take a step back and not rush to judgment about a patient's condition?

- This narrative reflects Rebecca's comfort in the clinical situation. How do you think you would have managed the push by the resident for the g-tube?

Listening Beyond the Yelling

Jesse MacKinnon, RN   **Practice level: Advanced Clinician**
Clinical Nurse, Oncology

John had an abusive father, an absent mother, and a diagnosis of pancreatic cancer at the age of 30. His cancer was complicated by a surgical scar that opened repeatedly and the ongoing development of fistulas that leaked bile into his stomach. This caused severe pain and left John with many tubes throughout his chest and abdomen.

John was angry. He had developed a reputation for yelling, swearing, and threatening staff. On my first day with John, he lived up to his reputation, calling me every name in the book. But something about him was likable. I saw he had a dry sense of humor. I knew I needed a way to establish trust so he'd feel comfortable enough to open up to me. John's primary concern was pain—he was receiving pain medication every 2 hours. His biggest fear was that his medication would be forgotten, and he would be left in unbearable pain. I made sure to bring John his pain medication every 2 hours, on the hour. This allowed him to feel more at ease. He even commented that I "cared about his pain as much as he did."

Over the next few weeks, John did open up to me. He talked about restaurants, fishing, and his favorite things in the world—his two dogs. Other than his sister, his dogs were the only living creatures he trusted. Overall, John was a sensitive, kind, caring person, but his severe pain and loss of hope and independence had masked those qualities. John didn't need antidepressants as some suggested; he needed a trustworthy friend, coach, and nurse. So that's what I set out to be.

During his months in the hospital I urged him to take walks, shower, and even be a little less harsh with staff. I walked with him, even after my shift ended, and I was always present when a doctor had to deliver bad news. I listened to him when he talked about his care, or when he just wanted to talk about a movie. We scheduled his 2-hour dressing changes for days when I was working. During those dressing changes, I focused on providing support and being totally present to him.

After a month and a half on our unit, John went home to be with his sister and his two dogs. Unfortunately he returned after a few weeks, this time with a systemic infection that was ravaging his body. John was in severe pain, couldn't eat, and had no quality of life to speak of. He confided in me that he was ready to die. All he wanted was to be comfortable and to no longer pursue treatment.

But John wasn't dying of cancer; it was the infection. Many of his doctors didn't want to give up. There was great disagreement among the team; some passionately wanted to try and save him, whereas others compassionately wanted to let him go.

I reminded them that John no longer wanted treatment. I called a meeting so the team could hear it directly from John. I arranged for John to meet with a representative from Patient Advocacy. At a second meeting, with my support, John explained why he no longer wanted to live "this life." The team finally understood. Treatment was stopped, and John spent a comfortable final 2 days with his sister and his beloved dogs.

This was a turning point in my career. John made me realize that true nursing isn't elaborate or complicated; it is simply understanding the needs of a fellow human being. It's about connecting with another person and trying to lessen his or her suffering. We all have times of anguish and pain. We all need someone to trust and rely on, to instill hope in us, and to connect to us on a basic human level. John showed me that true nursing care doesn't occur between a nurse and a patient—it occurs between people. John will remain in my heart as a constant reminder of why I became an oncology nurse.

Commentary

Short and simple, but oh, so powerful. Jesse saw beyond the anger and aggressive behavior to the vulnerable person who was his patient. He treated John with compassion and respect, and John responded in kind. Jesse's credibility with the rest of the team allowed them to also see John in a new light. Most important, Jesse's advocacy to end treatment allowed John to die peacefully, on his own terms, and in the company of his family and his beloved dogs.

Reflective Questions

- What have you seen in your patients that others did not see? How did you get others to see what you saw?

- How do you establish rapport and trust with a patient who is labeled as "difficult"?

- What can you do to advocate for a patient's wishes, even when the rest of the care team disagrees?

Step by Step

Janice Tully, RN
Case Manager, Cardiology

Practice level: Advanced Clinician

As the nurse case manager covering the Cardiac Intensive Care Unit (CICU) and the Cardiac Telemetry Unit, I am consulted for a variety of issues, including referrals to visiting nurse associations, rehabs, or hospice and transfers to other acute-care settings. I often meet with families at a time when their loved ones are critically ill to assist them in navigating the healthcare system. I do my best to support them in a safe transition of care.

One recent patient, Rosemary, whom I worked with on the Cardiac Telemetry Unit, was admitted for severe right-sided heart failure and acute worsening of her pulmonary hypertension. She was volume overloaded and needed diuresis. Although she had been followed in the Pulmonary Hypertension Clinic, her condition had deteriorated, and she was being evaluated for IV-Flolan. IV-Flolan is indicated for the treatment of pulmonary arterial hypertension to improve exercise capacity. Her past medical history was significant; she had endured a very long hospitalization and rehab stay in the recent past. She had been living on her own but recently moved into her sister's home to be closer to the hospital.

When I first met Rosemary, I saw a critically ill woman who was very guarded and barely made eye contact. She deferred my questions to her mother and sister, so I told her I'd be back when they were present. I understood she was tired from the admission process, and I encouraged her to rest—my assessment could wait. Over the next week, I got to know Rosemary and checked in with her daily. Prior to her becoming ill, she had enjoyed gardening and photography, but the progression of her medical issues had limited her ability to engage in these activities. Over the next 2 weeks, Rosemary's heart failure medications were carefully titrated, and she improved, gaining strength. When I came to see her, I was thrilled to see a smiling Rosemary ambulating in the hallway with her portable IV-Flolan at her side. Rosemary was at a point where she could begin to learn about the ambulatory fluid pump—CAAD, IV-Flolan mixing, and the care necessary to independently manage her medication at home.

IV-Flolan administration can be challenging. Patients need to be able to mix the drug daily, know how the CAAD pump works, and demonstrate the ability to troubleshoot and problem-solve as the half-life of the drug is less than 5 minutes. If therapy is interrupted, it can cause rebound hypertension and a potentially critical situation.

Rosemary was referred to a specialty pharmacy for help managing her medication at home. Teaching sessions offered by the pharmacy nurse were very focused and intense. I noticed that Rosemary was having trouble following along; the sessions weren't progressing as we had hoped. Many discussions followed to try to figure out the problem.

Rosemary said she was nervous about her mother, who was asking questions and trying to be part of the process. Other family members were present, as well, wanting to hear the teaching session and trying to be supportive. Despite several attempts at instruction, Rosemary struggled with the basic techniques. I conferred with her nurses to see if there would be a better time for teaching when she might be more able to absorb the material. We looked at factors such as the activity of a double room and the effect of her medications.

Our assessment was that her medications might be increasing her somnolence in the morning, so we asked her physician to adjust the medication regime accordingly. We restricted her teaching sessions to one-on-one with Rosemary and her nurse and provided a quiet room where they could talk without interruption. It seemed to help. Slowly, Rosemary began to make progress.

I shared with Rosemary an experience I had with another IV-Flolan patient who also felt frustrated and overwhelmed learning about the CAAD pump and mixing her medication. I assured her that the patient's anxiety had faded over time. It was like driving a car—after a while, the process would become second nature. I told her about a 17-year-old patient with a learning disability who had been able to learn the process and went on to go to her senior prom.

With encouragement and patience, Rosemary became more confident. Her physicians suggested that she go to rehab for continued teaching, as she wasn't quite able to manage in the home setting. She didn't have any physical or occupational therapy needs, so I advocated for her to be given more time to learn here. Rosemary had had a difficult time in the past with a long rehab stay, and she confided she didn't want to go back to rehab. Very few rehab facilities accept patients on IV-Flolan (I've only successfully moved one patient with IV-Flolan to a rehab setting). I agreed that it wouldn't be in Rosemary's best interest to go to rehab. I advocated for her to stay on the Cardiac Telemetry Unit until she was able to go directly to her sister's home. I reminded the team that Rosemary had been quite ill when she first arrived, which delayed initiation of her teaching sessions. After much discussion among the team, Rosemary's family, and me, we decided against a transfer to rehab.

Rosemary continued to improve with one-on-one teaching sessions. She got to know and trust the team on the unit. She became more focused and proficient at preparing her medications, and she practiced on her own throughout the day. Her confidence really started to emerge.

The home health nurse coordinated a predischarge visit to her sister's home to review things with the family. Before being discharged, Rosemary thanked me for my role in helping her get healthy and more comfortable with managing her healthcare needs.

I believe partnering with Rosemary, her family, the team, and the pharmacy was vital to her successful transition to her sister's home. Her hope was to return to her own home out of state after a period of time. I'm confident Rosemary has the ability and determination to live independently and will succeed in reaching that goal as well.

A follow-up call with Rosemary's nurse in the outpatient setting confirmed that she is managing quite well in her own home.

Commentary

Janice's experience with IV-Flolan and, more importantly, her knowledge of Rosemary had a profound effect on the outcome of this clinical situation. Janice recognized the stress Rosemary was feeling and the impact it had on her ability to process critical information. She worked with the rest of the team so that they also recognized that this was a problem that could be overcome. Janice's credibility with the team was clear as medications were adjusted and the discharge plan was changed.

Reflective Questions

- Janice advocated for many changes in Rosemary's treatment plan, such as her medication and the teaching plan. How would you get the team to buy into the plan?

- As a case manager, you know the pressure that surrounds discharging a patient home or to a rehab setting. When you advocate for a patient to stay in the hospital, how do you convince the team that this is the right course? What if they don't agree; what would you do?

- What have you learned about assessing the best way to teach patients and families this and other complex interventions they need to do at home?

Overcoming Fear

Julie MacPherson-Clements, RRT   **Practice level: Advanced Clinician**
Respiratory Therapist, Respiratory Acute Care

I immediately loved working in the Respiratory Acute Care Unit (RACU)—the interdisciplinary collaboration, the challenge to wean patients off ventilators, and the daily learning that comes with every patient assignment. Perhaps most important, I enjoy being able to engage patients in their own care because they're no longer sedated or on medication that limits their ability to participate in therapy.

Ellie had not sought medical care in more than 40 years and was admitted for shortness of breath. It was determined that she had a ruptured ulcer in the context of newly diagnosed chronic obstructive pulmonary disease (COPD). She had been intubated and extubated several times in the Surgical Intensive Care Unit (SICU). After long deliberations with her family, the decision was made to have a tracheostomy placed. Ellie's family had told the SICU team that being connected to a machine for the rest of her life would be an "albatross" to Ellie, who had effectively avoided medical care for the majority of her life. Knowing this, the team was even more determined to wean her off the ventilator.

When Ellie was admitted to the RACU, her daughter and sister accompanied her. I introduced myself and explained that my role was to help wean her from the machine and move her toward being able to talk with a trach. This would help her to be able to participate in physical therapy, speech therapy, and occupational therapy. Although her family's reaction was hopeful and optimistic at the progress she could make, Ellie's response seemed to be one of apathy. I imagined that with all she'd been through, hope was in short supply.

The next day, I started to wean Ellie from the ventilator after measuring some pulmonary mechanics on the ventilator. According to the numbers, she should have been able to breathe on her own. However, she expressed anxiety at the thought of doing any increased "work," despite insisting that she didn't want to be on a breathing machine for the rest of her life. Over the course of the next few days, Ellie was able to wean down to minimal settings, and it looked as if she was going to be able to breathe on her own. But after I took away the support of the machine to conduct a spontaneous breathing trial, her breathing pattern changed immediately. She started forcefully exhaling, had mono-phasic wheezing, and became highly anxious. I quickly put her back on the ventilator and stayed with her until her breathing was more comfortable.

Based on my observations, I asked the team to perform a bronchoscopy. I wanted to see if the trach tube was positioned correctly in her airway. If it wasn't, it could have been masked while she was on the ventilator, and then when the vent was taken away, her airway could have collapsed against the tube. I explained my theory to the team, and we immediately looked with the broncho-scope. I suggested we visualize the posterior wall of the trachea while Ellie was receiving positive pressure and then again without it. Sure enough, the tube was about 80% occluded, which explained the breathing pattern I had witnessed.

The fellow asked me which tube I thought would be best, and I suggested one with a smaller outer diameter to allow for potential phonation and one that would be long enough to bypass the area of collapse. Ellie was anxious about the procedure, so I recommended we not make any changes until her family arrived later that afternoon and could provide emotional support. As I had anticipated, Ellie's family was very supportive, and the tube was changed without incident.

My next goal was to evaluate Ellie for a speaking valve. Again, the numbers indicated she should be able to talk, but Ellie resisted. She couldn't give a reason why she didn't want to use the speaking valve, but she flat-out refused. In all my years in the RACU, I'd never seen a patient who was *able* to use the speaking valve but simply wouldn't do it. It's usually the opposite—patients feel they have less anxiety when they have a voice to communicate.

During my next shift several days later, I read in the notes that Ellie had not used the speaking valve at all. I started to think about what I could do to help her feel better about using her voice and understand the benefits of using the speaking valve. I contacted Ellie's speech language pathologist (SLP) and asked if she'd meet with Ellie, Ellie's nurse, and me to help Ellie understand how the speaking valve would allow her to communicate and eat and to help us under-stand what may have been contributing to Ellie's reluctance to use it. I scheduled the meeting for a time when Ellie's family could be present.

It was a wonderful, collaborative discussion. Ellie's family was very support-ive and grateful, saying, "Look at all these people who are here to help you; you should take advantage of them."

After we left the room, I asked the nurse if she thought consulting the psychi-atric clinical nurse specialist about employing relaxation techniques might help. I had worked with a number of COPD patients over the years but had never encountered anyone whose anxiety had halted their treatment to this degree. We consulted the psychiatric clinical nurse specialist, and she visited Ellie later that day. She guided Ellie through some relaxation techniques that Ellie found very helpful in managing her anxiety.

Soon, Ellie learned to tolerate the speaking valve and was able to remain off the ventilator. It was a complex situation that required a high level of collabora-tion among the interdisciplinary team. It made me realize the value of getting other clinicians involved in a patient's care.

This experience taught me a lot about my role as a member of the RACU team. I realized that even though I was disappointed with Ellie's initial response to my treatment interventions, it didn't have to limit her progress. I was able to recruit other members of the team to help work through the challenges. Having the support of my colleagues helped me gain a better understanding of the resources available to help ensure positive patient outcomes.

Commentary

Julie's knowledge and past experience are reflected in this narrative. The change in Ellie's breathing triggered Julie to recommend a bronchoscopy because she rec-ognized that the change in breathing pattern was related to a malpositioned tube. This embedded knowledge allowed for the team to quickly correct the problem.

It might have been easy to focus on Ellie's complex respiratory condition, but Julie saw Ellie holistically, and that approach was critical to Ellie's success-ful outcome. Julie tells us that Ellie had avoided receiving healthcare for many years, and this information allowed Julie to recognize an added level of fear as Ellie found herself in the acute care setting, with its inherent loss of control.

Ellie's long hospitalization had taken its toll on her, not only physically but also emotionally. She had lost faith that she could recover. In such a state, Ellie needed others to give her the confidence to know that she could recover. Julie's ability to pull the team together showed Ellie that they had faith in her, and that faith allowed Ellie to have faith in herself. This strategy gave Ellie the courage and faith in herself to use the speaking valve and to breathe off of the ventilator.

Reflective Questions

- Is malposition of trach tubes a common problem? How do you teach other members of the team when to suspect that this might be an issue?

- Ellie avoided receiving healthcare for 40 years. How would you develop a trusting relationship with such a patient?

- Julie credits not only Ellie and her family for this successful outcome, but also the team. What makes for a successful team?

Holding Off the Inevitable

Kristen Kingsley, RN   **Practice level: Advanced Clinician**
Clinical Nurse, Respiratory Acute Care

The Respiratory Acute Care Unit (RACU) is an 18-bed unit designed for the care of patients requiring focused pulmonary care and the care of patients with general medical diagnoses. Many of our patients stay for many weeks, and over that time we—nurses, physicians, and therapists—develop strong relationships with them and their families. Each patient affects us; Jack was one of those patients.

Jack was a 63-year-old gentleman who had idiopathic pulmonary fibrosis and was admitted to the Intensive Care Unit (ICU) from his home due to increasing O2 requirements and pneumonia. Jack's pulmonary fibrosis was so severe that he was listed for a lung transplant. After stabilizing in the ICU, he was transferred to the RACU for pulmonary management and monitoring.

As I received report on his fragile respiratory status, I also learned that Jack was viewed as a "difficult" patient. As I continued to listen to report, I chose not to focus on the label of being "difficult." Instead, I focused on how nurses need to tailor their approach to all patients to meet their needs and to develop what I know all patients need—trust in their nurse.

To develop trust, one needs to know one's patient. I learned that Jack had served in the military; he was not an emotional person. He had a tough, strong personality, which was at the core of military discipline and leadership. Taking his cue, I approached him in a calm, direct manner, assuring him that I would care for him in any way he needed. I answered his questions, and if I did not have the answer, I got him the answer in a timely, efficient manner. He responded to this approach, and as the day progressed he became more relaxed with me. I found that one way he would cope was through telling jokes. I would follow his cues and joke right back at him.

A source of great frustration for Jack was the diet the physicians had ordered for him. Jack had been a diabetic for several years and had a very specific regimen he followed, which was very different from the diet he was ordered to have while hospitalized. I recognized that this was about much more than the food—it was an issue of control. So much had been taken away from him; he needed to be able to order his own diet. I asked him if I could contact his endocrinologist so that he could have his diet and insulin regime faxed to the unit. He agreed, and together we wrote the email that Jack sent. When the diet arrived on the unit, I went over it with the RACU physicians and advocated for the changes. Jack was relieved and felt in control when the orders were changed and he could once again have a few extra Cheetos, his favorite snack. I felt a sense of accomplishment that this small intervention meant so much to him.

Jack struggled to stay optimistic, yet he recognized the irony that his good luck, receiving a lung transplant, would result from someone else having bad luck. He would comment, "I am either leaving here with lungs, or I am leaving here in a box." I would acknowledge what he was feeling, but I would also work to point out the positive—his supportive family and that his pneumonia was resolving. But that redirection did not last long, and I knew I needed to collaborate with other members of the team. I told Jack I wanted to invite the psychiatric clinical nurse specialist to meet with Jack to discuss techniques to reduce stress. He initially agreed, but hearing about therapeutic touch and relaxation techniques were perhaps too much, and he asked her to leave. I was still concerned and told Jack that as he prepared, both physically and emotionally, for what lay ahead, I wanted to make sure he knew he had resources and support. I spoke with the transplant team social worker to ensure that she further explore coping strategies that would support Jack through this time.

To help bring a sense of normalcy to what is an abnormal experience, the physical therapist and I moved Jack's stationary bike next to the window so he could, on his daily rides, look outside and enjoy the sunshine and sights. I also made sure that the daily newspaper and magazines that he enjoyed were readily available at his bedside, and I continued to try to keep up with him in telling jokes. I truly believe laughter is critical in promoting healing.

The long hospitalization weighed on him, and there were many days that he was emotionally and physically exhausted. I, again, stayed present with him and found ways to give him control and normalcy. One issue that frustrated him was disruption to his sleep. He complained that he was having difficulty sleeping because every time he rolled over in bed he would become entangled by the cardiac leads or be awakened by the blood pressure cuff inflating. I advocated for the team to have his cardiac monitor discontinued and to limit the number of times his vital signs were checked at night as a way to promote sleep. They agreed, and the quality of his sleep improved.

For patients awaiting transplant, all focus is on ensuring they remain as healthy as possible. An infection or an intubation can lower them on the transplant list. For a patient with pulmonary fibrosis, the chances of being intubated were high. I was committed that this would not happen, though one day I was not sure I could keep that commitment. Jack had become very anxious, and despite being on 100% oxygen, he was unable to maintain his oxygen saturation above 85% at rest and 70% with any exertion. I notified the team, gave him his Ativan, and stayed with him as the respiratory therapist adjusted his oxygen settings. Slowly his oxygen levels improved. I put a sign on the door asking that no one enter the room without first checking with me.

At this time I was once again approached by other nurses who questioned whether the best approach would be for Jack to be intubated. Watching him struggle to breathe and with oxygen levels that didn't immediately respond to interventions, when was the point that intubation would be the best approach? I had detailed in my notes interventions to calm Jack and allow him to respond to the changes in his oxygen settings, but I recognized that not everyone—nurses, physicians, and respiratory therapists—would have the same comfort level in waiting out an emergency situation. I continued to advocate for Jack to be given every chance not to be intubated so that he would remain high on the transplant list.

Jack's wife and three children would come and visit him, and even on his dark days, their presence would lighten his mood. It was difficult for them to visit, though. His wife lived in New Hampshire and worked full time so that they would have health insurance, and one daughter was pregnant with his first grandchild. The family members expressed their gratitude to all members of the team for being there for Jack when they could not be.

Days turned to weeks and then months as Jack, and the rest of the team, waited for the call saying that he was getting a new pair of lungs. As I prepared to be off for a week, I wondered whether the call would come. I wanted to be there when it came, but I knew he was in the capable hands of my colleagues. And, thanks to all our work together, Jack had not been intubated. While I was off, I received a call from a nurse on the unit telling me Jack was on his way to the OR to receive a new pair of lungs. I broke down in tears.

I visited him while he was in the ICU and again was impressed by his courage and determination. Several months later, a card arrived from Jack containing a picture of him holding his new granddaughter on his way home from rehab. His biggest fight was over, and he was heading home to the family he loved.

Commentary

On her first day with Jack, Kristen performed one of the most important and, at times, the most challenging interventions clinicians can do—she suspended judgment. She did not pay attention to the whispers that Jack was difficult; she committed to being open and building a relationship with Jack by getting to know him. She gently tested the use of humor. She recognized that his military background meant he liked order, answers, and a quick response. Kristen provided all of this, and a relationship was formed. The strength of that relationship supported Jack through many ups and downs as he awaited transplant.

Kristen, and the rest of the team, knew that in order to stay on the transplant list, Jack had to be as healthy as possible, which meant staying off the ventilator. In this narrative, Kristen's clinical knowledge and expertise, and her knowledge of Jack, allowed her to walk the thin line between intubation and exquisite clinical management.

Reflective Questions

- You are often told many things about your patients, which can influence your perceptions of them. How do you stop having others' opinions influence you?

- What is funny to one person might be viewed as disrespectful to someone else. What do you look for when you test the use of humor on a patient? How do you teach this skill to less-experienced nurses?

- Jack was awaiting a donor organ, which might or might not come. How do you balance giving such a patient hope with the reality of the situation?

Summary

In this chapter you have read narratives describing how clinicians leverage the strength of the team to achieve the best outcome for patients. While teamwork and collaboration are critical to safe and effective care, they can be challenging in the healthcare environment, with its inherent time pressures and stress.

Sharing narratives on this theme, from clinicians at all practice levels, creates opportunities to reflect on how a clinician "makes the case" to other members of the team and advocates and seeks out resources to build a team around the patient.

References

Institute of Medicine (2000). *To err is human: Building a safer health system*. Washington, DC: National Academics Press.

Institute of Medicine (2001). *Crossing the quality chasm: A new health system for the 21st century*. Washington, DC: National Academics Press.

Joint Commission on Accreditation of Healthcare Organizations (2008). Behaviors that undermine a culture of safety. *Sentinel Event Alert*, 40, 1–4.

Chapter 5
Theme of Practice: Movement

Through observation, palpitation, and touch, the therapist uses knowledge and skill to assess the patients' functional ability.

The Importance of Movement as a Theme of Practice

Following the initial development of the Clinical Recognition Program at Massachusetts General Hospital (MGH), members of the Professional Development Committee met with members of their respective disciplines to validate and amend the criteria to better reflect their discipline's practice. When members from Occupational Therapy and Physical Therapy met, for example, they discovered that, given the nature of their practice, another major theme emerged: movement. The Occupational Therapists and Physical Therapists found that movement was so prominent in the discussions, separate from clinical knowledge and decision-making, that they advocated that it be pulled out as a separate and unique theme.

Narratives—Entry Level of Practice

Entry or Advanced Beginner therapists are developing their skills in being able to facilitate the desired movement pattern, while being able to facilitate patients' functional activities. This requires them to understand, through consultation with more experienced colleagues, normal patterns and responses—versus the abnormal response—and the appropriate intervention to address them.

Narratives—Clinician Level of Practice

Competent or Clinician-level therapists effectively use their palpation and manual skills to facilitate the patient achieving the desired movement. They demonstrate confidence in their ability to translate what they are seeing and feeling into a diagnosis and treatment plan. The narratives allow for a more in-depth, detailed, and nuanced discussion.

Narratives—Advanced Clinician Level of Practice

With continued practice, reflection, and supervision, therapists at the proficient or Advanced Clinician level of practice are able to efficiently use their palpation and manual skills to select interventions and continuously adapt them to meet patients' changing motor responses. The therapists integrate information from their sensory, visual, and cognitive systems at an automatic level.

Narratives—Clinical Scholar Level of Practice

At the expert or Clinical Scholar level, the therapists have a highly refined ability to palpate, observe, and guide the patient at an intuitive and subconscious level. This allows for a high degree of treatment specificity and creativity. Their treatments are highly focused and designed. Their narratives allow for discussions that promote reflection and understanding of challenging patients, ethical situations, or system concerns.

The narratives that follow describe the movement theme of practice across the physical therapy and occupational therapy discliplines and across the four levels of expertise, as described in Chapter 1. The unbundling through reflective questions, which follows a brief commentary on the narrative, allows you to reflect on your own practice or that of a colleague.

Family First

Robert Dorman, PT   **Practice level: Clinical Specialist***
Physical Therapist

I first became aware of Brian during interdisciplinary rounds. Brian was a young man in his twenties who had fallen asleep at the wheel and crashed his car. He suffered a left olecranon (elbow) fracture and a traumatic amputation of his left leg below the knee. He'd had surgery 2 days before the debridement of his leg and placement of a vacuum-assisted closure dressing. The plan was to return to the OR in 2 days to reassess the leg and perform either a wound closure or an above-the-knee amputation.

Brian was in a lot of pain, which prompted the medical team to request holding off on physical therapy, but I knew it was important to examine him as soon as possible. I knew he had a long recovery ahead of him, and the chances of developing secondary problems (such as restricted range of motion in his knee) increased the longer that physical therapy was delayed. I could also provide some patient education that might alleviate concerns he had about the future. I discussed my reasoning with the medical team, and they agreed it was OK to proceed. I prepared for the examination.

I entered Brian's room, introduced myself, and explained why a physical therapist consult had been ordered. Brian was lethargic from pain medication but agreed to the exam. As we talked, I learned that Brian lived on his own and had a supportive family. He loved to ski and hike and described himself as a risk-taker. Brian co-owned a small business with his father, who had recently suffered a stroke. He became emotional as he worried aloud that the family business might not survive now that he had been injured, too. I could tell that this was a major source of stress for Brian that could potentially affect his progress if not addressed. I asked if he wanted to speak with a social worker, but he declined. This was something I'd need to monitor throughout his treatment. Given that Brian was in significant pain, I prioritized my exam. My main focus was positioning and range of motion of his injured left knee and hip. He had a pillow

---

*Because Robert Dorman is in the Clinical Specialist role in Physical Therapy, he is not eligible for the Clinical Recognition Program. Nonetheless, his narrative serves as an important lesson.

under his knee that caused it to flex about 30 degrees. I knew from research that knee-flexion contractures make using prosthesis more difficult, sometimes even impossible. To minimize the risk, I wanted to educate Brian about good positioning and give him some exercises that could help him keep his knee straight.

Shortly after I began, Brian said, "I might not even have a knee after tomorrow, why worry about it?"

I explained that the surgical plan was unknown, so we should hope for the best and try to preserve the knee. I showed him how to position the pillow to keep his knee straight and gave him some exercises to do throughout the day to help with his range of motion. Brian became so lethargic due to some of his medications that I decided to end the session. Before leaving, I asked if he had any questions. Most patients who've suffered a traumatic amputation have a lot of questions—I wanted to give him a chance to ask them if he had any. And he did. He asked about prosthetic options, functional outcomes, the rehab process, and more. I could tell it had been on his mind. As a physical therapist, I have the unique opportunity to bridge the medical condition and pathology with functional outcome. I feel privileged that I'm able to give patients information they want, especially related to function and ability to participate in activities.

Brian was young, had been active prior to the accident, had a good support system, and was highly motivated to get back to work. All of this worked in his favor. But he was also a risk-taker, which could increase his risk of falling and hinder his recovery. His elbow fracture meant no weight bearing on his left arm for at least 6 weeks. This, combined with his below-the-knee amputation, was going to make mobility a challenge. I knew the sooner Brian got a prosthesis, the better. Evidence suggests that a semi-rigid dressing on a residual limb has a number of benefits over soft dressings. Semi-rigid dressings protect the wound, minimize the knee-flexion contracture, help control edema, and decrease pain. And a semi-rigid dressing is removable, which enables the team to perform wound care.

I believed Brian was a candidate for an immediate postoperative prosthesis (IPOP). An IPOP is a temporary prosthesis that allows patients to begin gait training soon after surgery. Most IPOPs contain a semi-rigid dressing that becomes the internal socket of the prosthesis. This system achieves two important goals: The semi-rigid dressing protects the residual limb, and the temporary prosthesis allows the patient to mobilize sooner without having to use the upper extremities. Standard medical care is soft dressings. However, I strongly believed a semi-rigid dressing and IPOP system were what Brian needed, so I advocated for him to get them. I explained my rationale to the team, and they agreed. The next day, Brian went back to the OR, and the surgical team was able to close the wound, preserving the knee and maintaining the below-the-knee amputation. Afterward, I worked with Brian on keeping his knee extended. He preferred to have it flexed as it was more comfortable, so I came up with an idea that would help balance the time he spent with his knee extended and the time he spent in a position of comfort. Brian had not been able to mobilize, so I got a wheelchair and began transfer training. Not only did this help with positioning, but it also allowed him to leave the room and gave him a new sense of independence.

I contacted the prosthetist to coordinate my next PT session. Together, we assessed Brian's residual limb and confirmed he was a good candidate for an IPOP. Due to the location of the incision, however, he wouldn't be able to put it on until his wound healed. I still had concerns about Brian's penchant for risk-taking and wanted to get him into a semi-rigid dressing as soon as possible. Brian confided that he'd already lost his balance once, so time was of the essence.

The prosthetist and I educated Brian on the importance of protecting his residual limb. If he fell on it just once, he'd most likely destroy the muscle flap and need an above-the-knee amputation. I explained the difference between a below-knee and above-knee amputation in terms of functionality, but I got the sense Brian wasn't hearing me. I knew he was distracted by thoughts of his family and the struggle to keep the business going. Because of that, I stressed that injuring himself would result in more surgery, including, most likely, a higher amputation and a longer period of rehabilitation. He understood that meant not being able to provide for his family. With that, there was a definite change in Brian's attitude. He became very focused on our conversation.

Finally, he said, "My goal is to get better so I can take care of my family. I'll do whatever I need to do to be safe." He thanked me for being so direct with him and for helping him to see what he needed to do.

I followed Brian's progress throughout his hospitalization. Every time I saw him, I asked how his father was doing. I knew if he trusted me and saw I was invested in his success, he'd be more willing to accept my recommendations and actively engage in recovery. I believe every patient teaches us something. Brian taught me the importance of finding what's meaningful to each patient and incorporating it into the plan of care. Brian heard what everyone was saying to him; he just couldn't connect what we were telling him to his own situation. When I was able to link his desire to care for his family with the need to allow himself to heal (both physically and emotionally), he better understood the importance of being safe.

Brian experienced a traumatic event and has a long road ahead of him, but I'm confident my interventions helped speed his return to work and caring for his family, which was all that mattered to him.

Commentary

What a wonderful narrative of expert practice. Robert (Bob) is clearly present in the moment, but his skill and expertise allowed him to see the future when Brian will be walking, driving, and working and what Bob and Brian need to do to get there.

"Why bother?" was Brian's attitude. "Hope for the best," was Bob's. Without that early intervention—that preparation for the best-case scenario—Brian's story may have had a very different ending. Bob used one of the best tools any clinician has at his disposal: patient education. Bob gave Brian evidence-based information so that he could make an informed decision based on his own goals and priorities. Bob found what was meaningful for his patient and turned it into motivation to succeed.

Reflective Questions

- Therapists ask patients to begin the process of recovery when, despite medication, they can still be in pain. How do you approach patients to engage in treatment when they feel they cannot?

- Bob has to negotiate with Brian on his placement. How do you know when negotiating with a patient in the short run will allow for greater patient engagement in the future?

- Bob advocates for Brian to be considered for the IPOP. Have you advocated for a unique intervention for a patient because of the physical and emotional benefits it will have?

Learning From the Past

Vanessa Dellheim, PT   **Practice level: Clinician**
Physical Therapist

In physical therapy school, we are taught to assess impairments, distinguish functional limitations, and provide treatment to improve mobility. A few thoughts about this model come to mind with a particular patient of mine named Angelo.

Angelo was a 90-year-old male admitted after being found on the floor of his bathroom. In the emergency department, he was found to have had a myocardial infarction as well as bilateral subdural hematomas. Angelo lived with his wife, who suffered from dementia, in a two-family home. His son lived downstairs and told us that his father was independent in all activities of daily living. Angelo's past medical history also included Alzheimer's disease. Physical Therapy was consulted to assess safe mobility.

The initial evaluation was particularly difficult because Angelo responded to some commands; however, "open your eyes" was not one of them. He demonstrated tangential speech—"Yahoo! Move the red ones; take the blues ones over there."

He had impaired range of motion and gait. I anticipated additional impairments in sensation, muscle performance, and balance, but those things were difficult to assess because of Angelo's inability to follow commands.

During Angelo's initial evaluation, he required assistance for mobility second to unsteadiness as well as cognition. This acute decompensation was initially attributed to his subdural hematoma; however, after a few days there was no change in his performance. Understanding his baseline as explained by his son, I thought that with continued intervention and healing from his subdural he would progress toward his baseline. Unfortunately, this was not the case.

Angelo remained a patient on the general medical unit for 6 weeks, where I worked with him on balance and gait training. I tried many different activities to provide an effective treatment; however, difficulties arose due to his waxing and waning mental status. He did not respond to formal commands, but I found he did respond to more informal communication such as, "Let's go," and "Time to get up." I found changing my communication with him improved his interaction with physical therapy. One technique that proved to be effective was having him push a cart up and down the hallway. His son had informed me that he previously worked on a loading platform for the post office and was pushing and pulling bins every day, hence the meaning of his frequent statements of, "Bring the red ones over; no, the blue; I need 1, 4, and 5." I thought up and trialed treatments that would engage Angelo, such as pushing carts, stacking boxes, playing catch, and gait training while carrying objects and stepping over objects.

During his length of stay, while I was searching for effective treatments, I questioned whether there would be any carry-over even if I could consistently engage him. Despite knowing the progressive nature of dementia, I wondered whether, with repetition, implicit learning could be achieved. Research articles were inconclusive about the effects of exercise in dementia patients, which then prompted me to seek my clinical specialist guidance. We determined that optimizing Angelo's environment to promote adherence and cooperation with physical therapy should be the first step.

I realized Angelo's cognition and mental status were "driving the show"; however, we wondered whether we as a team could create a structured environment in which he would thrive (decrease agitation and improve function). Despite some improvement in mobility, Angelo still was unsafe to return home due to cognitive deficits, such as problem-solving, memory, and recognition of objects. During his time as a patient, I felt as though I became one of the constants compared to the revolving physicians, nurses, and aides in Angelo's life.

As Angelo's progress reached a plateau, I was not yet ready to discharge him. I was uncertain what other role I could take in his care. Soon I realized it was advocating for him. I began looking at him as the constant and looking at the staff and his environment as variables. Besides the actual one-to-one treatment time I spent with Angelo, I also spent time educating the nurses and the patient-care assistants on the best ways to approach him. I wanted to allow him to mobilize in a safe environment as well as manage his agitation. Through multiple discussions with the nurse practitioners, the nursing staff, and patient-care associates, we created an appropriate sleep/wake cycle utilizing the shades and initiated a toileting schedule to improve Angelo's quality of life and decrease episodes of incontinence. I also advocated for Angelo by initiating a discussion about the best long-term placement for him. I felt strongly that a structured dementia unit would be most effective at managing his behavior while still allowing him to thrive.

Eventually, Angelo's medications were managed so that he was alert and awake without significant agitation. The toileting schedule was effective but unfortunately did not correlate to fewer attempts to get out of bed. The nurses and aides enforced the bed/chair alarm and were able to redirect him by taking him for walks in the hallway. He was able to ambulate with supervision, which he required for safety. His reevaluations week to week had come to plateau. At this time, I realized I had challenged Angelo's balance and gait as best as he was able. In consultation with the clinical specialist, it was decided further training would need to be specific to his environment upon discharge. The next step, which was difficult for me, was to discharge him from the Physical Therapy service.

Angelo taught me that, as a physical therapist on an interdisciplinary team, there is more included in my practice than just treating a patient. I have recognized the importance of advocating for patients, especially the ones who are unable to speak for themselves. After treating Angelo, I began to not just look at the patient as a whole, but also to include the patient's environment and staff members. Treatment includes facilitating the appropriate environment and care of a patient throughout disciplines.

Commentary

Vanessa was unfazed by Angelo's age, dementia, complex medical history, and social circumstances. Her only thought was to help him achieve the highest level of functioning he could attain. She did that and more. She tailored her interventions to meet his processing requirements given his cognitive status. Vanessa skillfully identified how to create a safe plan to get him mobile by re-creating his past work experience. She became his advocate, ensuring that all members of the team "knew him" and knew how to approach him to optimize his care. She recognized the limits of physical therapy and created a plan and team to help Angelo hold on to the gains he had made.

Reflective Questions

- Patients' performance can fluctuate. How do you assess the best timing for physical therapy or other activities to maximize results?

- Vanessa utilizes various cues—visual, verbal, and tactile—in her work with Angelo. How do you determine which cues or combination of cues work best for a patient?

- Despite having a plan in place, discharging a long-term patient can be difficult. Can you describe a situation where you were faced with this issue? What made it difficult, and what did you learn from that experience?

Finding Jimmy

Jennifer McAtee, OTR/L
Occupational Therapist

Practice level: Advanced Clinician

I met Jimmy for the first time 2 days after he was admitted for a left-sided embolic stroke. He was 65 years old. After reviewing his chart, I learned he'd scored an 8 out of 42 on his National Institutes of Health Stroke Scale (NIHSS). Though a score of 8 is low, it's not a reliable predictor of function post-stroke. His follow-up head imaging report showed a hemorrhagic conversion of his stroke, so I knew through my education and experience I could anticipate more prominent neurological impairment.

I made a mental list of impairments I could expect to encounter during my evaluation, including impaired communication, apraxia, and right-sided motor and sensory impairments. I've learned that patients affected by left middle cerebral artery (MCA) strokes can demonstrate variable levels of functioning that don't correspond with traditional neurological assessment. Experience has taught me to use activities-of-daily-living (ADL) tasks during my evaluation to highlight potential impairments and establish an appropriate intervention plan. Left MCA strokes can affect the ability to comprehend verbal and written information and the ability to verbally express information. Patients with expressive language impairments often exhibit some impairment in receptive language, and I anticipated that might be the case with Jimmy.

Research suggests that in left MCA strokes, motor apraxia often reaches the right side of the body. Patients with ideational apraxia often reach for the wrong object, such as a comb to brush their teeth, or they demonstrate clumsy motor patterns, such as being unable to rotate a hairbrush appropriately. These patients may appear to "neglect" the affected side because it's too difficult to formulate or perform the movements required. So the patient simply doesn't use that side of the body.

I made a plan to engage Jimmy in three common tasks: combing his hair, putting on pants, and putting on socks. I chose these tasks because even if he exhibited receptive communication impairment, I'd be able to demonstrate what I was asking him to do.

As an occupational therapist, I rely heavily on information known as an *occupational profile* to learn how an individual's prior roles, routines, and daily contexts are affected by his or her illness or injury. There was very little documentation about Jimmy's social history or prior function. The only information I had was that he was right-hand dominant and lived with his niece. Jimmy's nurse reported that he was neglecting his right side. I was starting to build an understanding of who Jimmy was prior to his stroke and what kind of impairments he was exhibiting even before I entered his room.

When I met Jimmy, he was lying on his back against the bed rails on the right side of the bed. His sheets were tangled in his legs, and the right side of his hospital gown had fallen off his shoulder. He appeared somewhat guarded when I sat in the chair beside him, but he was willing to engage with me. I wanted to ensure that I had a basic understanding of any communication impairments he might have so that I could establish an effective mode of communication.

After introducing myself and my role, I asked Jimmy to perform some basic commands to ensure that he understood me. I asked questions that could be answered by nodding "Yes" or shaking the head "No," as research shows this to be an effective way to communicate with impaired communication. For non-Yes/No questions, I provided options, interpreted his gestures, and validated the information back to him. The fact that he was able to communicate beyond a simple Yes or No showed me that Jimmy was able to integrate all the things I was saying, and it gave me a way to establish a rapport with him by allowing us to communicate with one another.

As I continued to ask questions about his life, he grew more relaxed; he smiled when communicating about his likes and interests, he made eye contact, and he even gestured for me to sit beside him. All these nonverbal signs affirmed that we had begun to develop a level of trust. I learned that Jimmy lived with his niece in a walk-up apartment and that she worked full-time. He had retired within the last year and liked to eat out. He drove when needed, but preferred to walk when he could. I soon learned that Jimmy was actually left-dominant for all tasks except writing. He conveyed that he had learned to write with his right hand in elementary school when a teacher made him sit on his left hand.

Knowing Jimmy's dominance was key in engaging him in activities of daily living. Occupational therapists use activity-analysis to break down functional tasks to accurately identify any neurological impairment. Learning that Jimmy was naturally left-dominant changed the lens through which I would assess his performance. I could anticipate that he'd perform right-handed tasks with more difficulty, regardless of any motor impairment he may exhibit.

I felt I had the appropriate context to assess Jimmy's level of functioning. In observing him perform tasks such as dressing and hair combing, I noted he acknowledged his right upper extremity consistently, but required intermittent cues to engage it. He appropriately chose a comb for the task, but after he was finished he kept the comb in his hand while reaching for socks. His movements were clumsy and inaccurate, which frustrated him. He attempted to hold garments with ineffective grasps, and his right hand was notably worse than his left. Each time his dominant left upper extremity crossed the midline of his body, his motor performance and control of his arm deteriorated.

I combined these observations with the data I had gathered during my evaluation that showed Jimmy had intact strength, coordination, and sensation. My analysis revealed two important findings. First, based upon my understanding of neuroanatomy, I knew it would be very rare for him to demonstrate right spatial or body neglect. And second, right spatial or body neglect doesn't exist in conjunction with functional communication impairments because those two neurological deficits are housed in opposite hemispheres of the brain. Because I knew that Jimmy's stroke damage was limited to the left hemisphere, I felt confident that it wasn't right neglect he was exhibiting but motor apraxia.

After completing Jimmy's evaluation, it was clear he'd require further rehabilitation of his motor apraxia and communication impairments. Jimmy's prior level of independence, motivation to improve, and cognitive status told me he had an excellent chance at full recovery. I collaborated with his physical therapist and speech–language pathologist to ensure we were in agreement about his post-hospital rehabilitation needs. We agreed Jimmy should be discharged to an acute rehabilitation program. I gave his nurse some suggestions on how to assist Jimmy with daily self-care, including verbal reminders to use both hands during tasks and placing the spoon or fork in his left hand with a normal grasp at mealtime.

After identifying Jimmy's primary neurological impairments, I formulated a treatment plan with short-term goals focused on ADL tasks. I integrated verbal and tactile cues to facilitate motor planning of his upper extremities. Jimmy showed improvement in his motor planning and was able to feed himself independently with his dominant left hand by the end of our second treatment session. His progress not only confirmed the effectiveness of the treatment intervention but also facilitated a level of independence for Jimmy that he hadn't experienced since the stroke.

Gathering accurate information from Jimmy's occupational profile allowed me to employ an advanced evaluation process and accurately interpret the results. By integrating my knowledge of the information with my observations of his functional performance, I was able to tailor my evaluation method to incorporate the information he gave me about his left-hand dominance. This allowed me to create the most effective plan to facilitate his recovery.

Commentary

Jennifer's narrative beautifully captures her assessment of the physiological changes caused by Jimmy's stroke, and she efficiently anticipates the impact those changes would have on his ability to function in his daily life. Jennifer identified potential limitations and predictors of recovery through stroke scores and exams and then integrated those findings into her own evaluation using Jimmy's occupational profile. Jimmy recognized Jennifer as a partner on his road to recovery. The trust they established was key to Jennifer learning about his true dominance, which ultimately enabled her to craft a meaningful, effective plan of care for him. This is a wonderful example of the importance of "knowing" your patient.

Reflective Questions

- Jennifer's assessment showed that what appeared to be right-sided neglect was in fact a motor apraxia. Has your assessment ever changed a diagnosis of a patient? How did that new diagnosis impact your treatment interventions?

- Jennifer's discovery that Jimmy was naturally left-handed "changed the lens" through which she assessed and treated him. Have you ever cared for a patient where new information changed the lens through which you saw or treated the patient?

- How do you select an activity that challenges the patient but does not frustrate him or her?

The Occupation of Children

Sharon Serinsky, OTR/L   **Practice level: Advanced Clinician**
Occupational Therapist

Harry was a 3-year-old boy who was referred to Occupational Therapy following a neuro-psychological evaluation that showed some potential sensory-processing issues. The day before Harry's visit, I called his mother to learn more about him. She reported that he had difficulty self-regulating and had a low tolerance for change. I reviewed his medical record and found that Harry had recently been diagnosed with autism spectrum disorder and speech-language delays.

On the day of his visit, I greeted Harry and his parents and escorted them to the treatment room. My goal for evaluation was to help Harry become comfortable in the testing area. As he wandered around the room looking at the toys, his parents told me he enjoyed physical play with his father, but had difficulty interacting with unfamiliar people.

I explained that pediatric occupational therapy often looks like play. This is an important concept to understand because play is the occupation of children. Most everyone becomes motivated to try new activities that are perceived as fun.

Harry wasn't interested in playing with toys, and he didn't easily make eye contact. As we progressed through the evaluation, Harry insisted on not sitting at the table and climbed onto his father's lap. Though Harry had been referred for suspected sensory-processing issues, he was exhibiting other challenging behaviors, such as limited attention span, avoidance of tasks, frequent whining vocalizations, and limited social interaction. These behaviors can have a significant impact on the development of social, educational, and self-care skills. My objective was to determine which sensory issues were contributing to Harry's developmental delays and gain information about his responses to sensory input, his strengths and weaknesses, and his interactions with his parents.

A well-accepted sensory-integration theory is referred to as "top-down, bottom-up inhibition." It purports that the top part of the brain is used for cognitive thinking functions, whereas the bottom and back of the brain are responsible for regulating arousal levels through muscle and joint stimulation. I surmised that engaging Harry in an activity that provided "bottom-up inhibition" would move him into a more optimal state of self-regulation and provide calming sensory input.

As Harry continued to cling to his father, I introduced some soft theraputty, similar to Play-Doh or children's clay. Most 3-year-olds are familiar with it and enjoy manipulating it. Harry used only his fingertips, not his whole hand, to mold the putty, which suggested an over-sensitivity to touch input.

Next, I introduced a plastic accordion tube that provided a type of tactile or sensory input known as *tactile* or *proprioceptive* input. When manipulated, the toy provides resistance to movement and sensory input to the muscles and joints. This provides information about body awareness and the ability to detect speed, force, and direction of movement. Harry required hand-over-hand assistance to manipulate the tube, which he tolerated well; his vocalization decreased, and his whole body calmed. Most 3-year-olds have enough hand strength to push and pull the accordion tube independently. Harry didn't.

I introduced a medium-sized therapy ball, as Harry's father had reported that he enjoyed active play. Harry allowed me to place him on the ball and bounce him up and down gently. He allowed me to move him slightly side-to-side and back-and-forth. Again, the activity calmed him and led to a decrease in his vocalizations.

As I introduced other activities, I continued to gather information about Harry and his sensory processing. He tolerated slow, linear movements when suspended on a piece of equipment, but became upset if his feet didn't touch the mat. He resisted changes in body and head position. These responses indicated gravitational insecurity, another sign of difficulty with sensory processing of movement and sensory integration.

Though I was unable to complete an extensive evaluation, I was able to identify Harry's strengths and weaknesses and develop an initial course of treatment. One of my goals was to assist Harry's parents to understand and observe his sensory-motor needs as a first step toward sensory integration treatment. Harry's parents were able to implement simple sensory activities at home that helped prepare and familiarize Harry with activities we'd be doing in treatment.

Going forward, I changed the way I prepared the environment and myself for Harry's visits. I reduced visual distractions and prepared materials to minimize disruptions in the flow of treatment. I soon realized that planning fewer activities was better suited to Harry's ability to process sensory input. I applied this same principle to the way I interacted with Harry. I increased the time it took to go from the waiting area to the treatment room, spending more time talking with his parents in order to reassure Harry. I began using the same activity at the beginning of every session, which enabled Harry to transition more easily. As I approached treatment at a slower pace, my own interactions slowed down as well.

By the fourth session, Harry was becoming more comfortable and began to participate more actively in treatment sessions. While he continued to jump in place and appear anxious in the waiting area, he was eager to go to the treatment room as he visually recognized me. I actively incorporated his parents into our activities, which was reassuring to Harry and helped reduce his need to constantly check in with them. I began to incorporate music into the sessions, singing familiar songs to him. This was also calming and brought out Harry's sense of humor—he would laugh when I purposefully sang the wrong words, which he would eventually correct. Harry became more joyful during treatment. His eye contact increased, and he was more easily engaged to work on fine-motor tasks such as stringing beads and learning to cut with scissors. One of the goals of sensory-integration treatment is to provide the child with just the right amount of challenge to enable him to develop skills and self-confidence.

Harry's progress was a combination of strong parental involvement to ensure carry-over and support of treatment goals and direct occupational therapy. My role was to empower Harry's parents to become active participants in the treatment process in the clinic as well as at home. My goal was to help Harry integrate sensations more appropriately so he could engage in adaptive responses and have more success mastering the developmental tasks of childhood. The process will be ongoing for Harry and his family. Harry needs to have more successes in order to feel comfortable and take on new challenges. My goal as a therapist will be to guide him through this process.

Commentary

In this narrative we see Sharon's keen sense of observation and analysis as she integrated Harry's response to touch and activity and shifted her interactions in response. Each toy she gave Harry was a deliberate choice for assisting her in the evaluation process. She was comfortable in evaluating and treating children with the diagnosis of sensory-processing issues and mindful and deliberate in her use of touch with Harry. Too much and his reaction would stop the evaluation process; too little and she would not be able to truly evaluate his body's response.

Reflective Questions

- Family involvement is key to ensuring that the treatment plan is continued at home. How do you assess families' readiness to participate? How do you build their observation and palpation skills?

- As a patient progresses in treatment, how do you begin to identify long-term goals? How do you know those goals are realistic and achievable?

- Integration of "bottom-up" and "top-down" components into the treatment plan requires skill and knowledge of the patient. How do you know how and when to integrate such an approach to a treatment plan?

Writing a New Chapter of a Life

Kim Erler, OTR/L   **Practice level: Advanced Clinician**
Occupational Therapist

I have been an occupational therapist for 2½ years. The day I met John started no differently from any other Monday. As I started to read about new patients who had been admitted over the weekend, a nurse came to ask me about the care plan for one of her patients. It was then that I learned about John, a 20-year-old student who had fallen 4 stories and sustained a C6 spinal-cord injury and bilateral wrist fractures.

After my initial heartbreak for a patient I had yet to meet, I started to think about what my role would be and the best time to initiate occupational therapy. I wasn't intimidated by the severity and complexity of John's injuries; I was excited about this opportunity to work with him in the acute phase of injury. I knew how important occupational therapy would be for his long-term success and functional recovery.

As a student, I had completed a 3-month clinical rotation at a rehabilitation hospital working on the adolescent and young adult team. During that time, I developed a passion for working with individuals whose lives had been changed by spinal-cord injuries. I love that those unique skills of occupational therapy can help patients who've had everything taken away from them to regain control of their lives. After doing a quick "walk-by" of John's room, I realized that translating what I had learned into the rehab setting to the acute-care experience would make for an interesting challenge given the fragility of his medical status at this stage.

Although John's medical status was tenuous, it was clear that occupational therapy should be initiated as soon as possible. John's spinal cord was damaged at the C6–7 level, meaning he could move his arms, shoulders, and elbows, but his wrists would be much weaker, and his digits might not have any active movement at all. Being able to move his wrists would be essential if he hoped to participate in functional tasks using what's called a *tenodesis grasp*. Evaluating John's strength was going to be difficult because he was in heavy postoperative "casts" that restricted his movement. I decided a conversation with the orthopedic service was warranted to discuss his orthopedic precautions in the setting of his neurological rehab.

After much discussion about what was best for John, the orthopedic doctor agreed that he should be placed in lightweight splints and permitted to do gentle range-of-motion exercises. It was time to execute the plan and begin rehabilitation.

When I went to meet John for the first time, he was still on a ventilator, which made communication very difficult. I explained I was part of the rehab team and that my role was to help him start participating in his self-care again. He appeared disinterested, keeping his eyes closed, until I removed the heavy post-op casts, and then he briskly raised both arms with an ear-to-ear grin.

During the next few sessions, we focused on moving and strengthening his arms. He was consistently demonstrating a return to C7, which meant he was able to straighten his arms and extend his wrists. Although that might not seem any more important than any other movement, I knew that the ability to extend arms might mean that he might eventually be able to transfer himself. And being able to extend his wrists would give him the tenodesis grasp, which meant he would be able to perform his activities of daily living (ADLs) independently.

One day John kept trying to tell me something, but I just couldn't read his lips. Finally, his mother said, "Are you trying to say you want to look outside?" And with a nod of his head that couldn't be misinterpreted, John's message was clear. The ICU nurses, who never fail to go above and beyond for their patients, worked together to rearrange his bed, ventilator, and other equipment so John could look outside. It was clear to me that the architectural design of the Lunder building had a visible impact on this young man's rehab. He was able to exert control over his environment when control over everything had been taken away. To me, this was about much more than being able to look outside. It was about John taking the first step in advocating for his own needs. This was a pivotal moment in his rehab. It told me he was ready for more. Because John was an amateur writer and constantly frustrated by not being able to speak (despite becoming proficient in adaptive strategies like the communication letter board),

I chose writing as one of his treatment options. I thought it would be a meaningful and motivating activity for him, and he might be able to achieve some success at it. I also thought that being able to brush his own teeth would help motivate him to want to engage in his own ADLs again.

A *universal cuff* is a piece of equipment that wraps around a person's palm and has an insert into which tools can be placed. It allows people who don't have the ability to activate their digits to "hold" items. When I entered John's room, I asked if he'd like to try these activities, and he immediately spelled out the word "No" on his letter board. He went on to spell the word "Normal." John didn't want to do anything if he couldn't do it the way he had before his injury.

Expecting him to be reluctant, I gave him the option of writing or brushing his teeth. He chose writing. I placed the universal cuff on his left hand because it was slightly stronger, and I inserted the pen. In very short order, John wrote his name. He smiled. I smiled. His mom smiled so hard she cried. John kept at it, eventually writing, "I'm right-handed. Can we put it in the other hand?" John had real success writing. I wanted to push him to brush his teeth, but he was too tired. When I left, he agreed to try to brush his teeth with his nurse that night. The next day, his nurse found me to tell me he'd done a great job and that he'd been the one to remind *her* that *he* was supposed to try it himself. The positive reinforcement of being successful at writing had given him the confidence to try another adaptive task. I rarely choose writing as the first task for a person with a new spinal-cord injury, but for John it was just right because it was motivating and important to him.

I became an occupational therapist because I wanted to make a difference in people's lives by facilitating participation in meaningful activities. John was just at the beginning of his journey. And it was clear he would have many more bumps along the road to recovery. But in the state-of-the-art ICU room with John's bed facing out the window, I know I made a difference helping him get some independence back.

A few weeks later, John was transferred to rehab at the same facility where I had done my clinical rotation as a student. I'll never forget my sessions with John because that experience made me a better clinician.

Commentary

Kim's narrative gives us insight into the intricate planning that goes on before an occupational therapist even enters the patient's room—understanding the back story and the effect the injury will have on a patient's life, as well as the many complexities of the injury itself. When Kim entered John's room with that universal cuff, it could have gone either way. But Kim made the session meaningful for John by quickly readjusting the cuff to maximize not only his hand movement, but also to give John an opportunity to regain some control over his life.

Kim's passion for working with individuals whose lives are changed by spinal-cord injuries was clearly evident in this narrative.

Reflective Questions

- How have your past experiences, in school or in a work setting, informed your practice? What are the challenges associated with translating those past skills to your current practice setting?

- The ability to engage with a patient in his or her recovery requires that the patient find meaning in the activity. How does your knowledge of the patient inform the activity you use in treatment?

- Kim utilizes the universal cuff to allow John to write. Have you had a patient where the activity challenge exceeds the patient's activity?

Moving Past the Pain

Alyssa Evangelista, PT **Practice level: Clinical Scholar**
Physical Therapist

Through educational opportunities and my practice, I've become more adept at evaluating and treating complex medical conditions and managing the socio-economic needs of my clients. I've learned to treat each patient as a "whole person," using connections within the community and the healthcare center to provide the best possible care.

One patient, Anna, was an 88-year-old woman I've treated through two episodes of care for orthopedic conditions. I had worked with Anna's son and granddaughter, as well as her late husband. Anna presented with complaints of acute exacerbation of chronic lower-back pain. Like many patients, Anna had numerous other medical and social concerns, as well.

Anna's husband had passed away suddenly a few months before. They'd been married more than 60 years, and she had been devoted to him. Anna had a history of vertigo, bilateral hearing loss, low blood pressure, vertebral artery aneurysm, and extensive, degenerative joint disease.

During my initial evaluation, Anna reported a high level of pain (10 out of 10) and disability. She said she was primarily limited in her ability to ambulate or stand for any length of time, which kept her from baking (her favorite hobby). She perceived the pain as caused by her spine and found it devastating and disabling. I delved into the social and emotional challenges she'd gone through since the death of her husband. She revealed that she hadn't been leaving the house much. Prior to her husband's death, she'd attended exercise classes at a senior center, but due to transportation issues and sadness, she hadn't been able to go back there. Anna shared that her daughter would be retiring soon, and she'd be able to spend more time with her out in the community after that happened.

Due to her reported pain, I had to rule out any pathological causes. Anna is an older, thin, Caucasian woman with a history of osteoporosis, so I was concerned it could be a vertebral stress fracture, but her physician had ordered imaging, which revealed no fracture. It did reveal a severely degenerated lumbar and thoracic spine with marked curvature causing scoliosis. Due to the amount of degeneration, my assessment veered away from stress fracture; Anna's complaints were more consistent with arthritic symptoms. Because Anna's pain was mechanical versus pain that doesn't change with motion or repositioning, I felt confident her degenerative changes were the primary cause of her dysfunction.

I was also concerned about Anna's balance, so I performed some tests to determine whether she was at risk for falling. Anna had lost considerable strength in her legs and trunk muscles. She had multiple areas of bilateral, lower-extremity muscle shortening and hypo-mobility throughout her lumbar spine. Testing showed a loss of protective reflexes and balance while walking or ambulating on uneven surfaces. Her sensory testing was normal. During Anna's history and evaluation, it became clear that her pain had a strong emotional component. She had become depressed as well as deconditioned (her physical strength had weakened). I knew from working with Anna before that when educated on causes and treatment of injuries, she reported lower levels of pain and disability. I had to not only verbally explain my findings, but also use visual tactics and meaningful examples. I showed Anna the images of her spine compared to images of a normal, healthy spine. I used a model to demonstrate how compression from advanced arthritis can cause lower-extremity symptoms and pain.

We discussed realistic, outcome-based goals. I paid special attention to the activities Anna felt caused her pain and disability, including baking, walking, and house cleaning. I instructed Anna that she'd need to change her body mechanics to protect her lumbar spine and that because of her arthritic changes, the long-term outcome would not be 100% resolution. She'd need to be proactive in managing her arthritis to prevent flare-ups. Anna had felt isolated since the death of her husband. Realizing that socialization and outside activities were important, I discussed ways to re-integrate her into the community. I'm active in the senior wellness group at the health center, and I felt the program would be an excellent fit for Anna because it encompassed social, medical, and general well-being initiatives. Anna thought it was a great idea and looked forward to working out with people her age.

During subsequent visits with Anna, I used manual therapy to address her pain, and I addressed her balance issues with manual and visual feedback. I gave Anna a home exercise program, which we practiced together to make sure she was doing it correctly.

After three follow-up visits, Anna continued to complain of low-back pain at a 10/10 level. She would experience temporary improvement after manual therapy for about 48 hours. I realized she'd need more manual therapy, strength, and endurance training to see real gains in her pain and function. Anna, however, was upset that she didn't feel better. We decided to explore other options for pain control until Anna was stronger and more flexible.

I spoke with Anna and her daughter about the use of heating pads and Lidoderm patches. We discussed when and how long to apply them and how to prevent skin irritation. I suggested bracing her spine during extended periods of standing and housework. We tried a standard lumbar support, but Anna didn't have the upper body strength to put it on and take it off. After a little brainstorming, we decided to try a girdle she had at home. Anna had used this girdle to manage her pain before. I cautioned her that the girdle was only a temporary method, and she shouldn't become dependent on it.

Anna soon began to report a significant and lasting decrease in her level of pain. By now, Anna's daughter had retired and was able to spend more time with her. We developed a plan to promote endurance and combat feelings of social isolation by walking in the mall and visiting friends. Anna also started to participate in tai chi and yoga classes at the health center. Because Anna's pain was better controlled, I switched my focus from manual therapy and pain management to strength and endurance training and balance retraining.

During Anna's final visits, she reported 1 or 2 days of increased pain, but she was much more adept at employing strategies to control it. She realized that if she addressed her pain early and modified her body mechanics, she could prevent high levels of pain for an extended period of time. Anna ended her physical therapy treatment with a good plan for long-term pain management and an exercise program that promoted maintenance of her strength and function.

During my continuing education as a physical therapist, I've learned that the best outcomes are achieved when we work together with our patients and families as a team. Using resources available in the community and throughout MGH, I'm able to promote health and wellness for patients like Anna during their episodes of care and for long-term well-being.

Commentary

It's significant that Alyssa showed equal concern for Anna's physical and emotional well-being. Both had a bearing on her recovery. In this narrative we see Alyssa's highly refined skill of palpation, guidance, and knowledge of movement. There are no wasted steps. Alyssa was candid with Anna about the long-term effects of arthritis, but at the same time, Alyssa educated and empowered Anna to take control of her pain management through exercise, socialization, and medication. Alyssa used a multifaceted approach to meet Anna's physical, emotional, and psychosocial needs and help facilitate her re-entry into the community.

Reflective Questions

- Many patients hope or expect that therapy will end their pain rather than manage it. How do you work with patients to understand that they will not be pain free?

- Alyssa's exam identified multiple factors contributing to Anna's balance problems. When a patient's exam identifies multiple problems, how do you prioritize those issues to develop a safe and effective plan?

- How does a patient's age have an impact on when and how you use manual therapy?

Summary

The work of the clinical disciplines requires clinicians to be guided in their interventions not only by data and metrics but also by reading and understanding what the patient is saying or not saying, and what is occurring or what is not and should be. In this chapter, occupational and physical therapists have shared their narratives on how the knowledge gained through touch and observation allows them to understand what is happening inside the complex systems of the body and through this knowledge intervene to ensure the best outcome for the patient.

References

Jensen, G., Gwyer, J., Hack, L., & Shepard, K. (2007). *Expertise in physical therapy practice.* Philadelphia, PA: Saunders Elsevier.

Chapter 6

Strategies to Hardwire a Narrative Culture

We hope that the previous chapters have given you insight into how the use of clinical narratives can assist clinicians in the development of a reflective practice, make their practice more visible, identify barriers to excellent practice, and showcase best practice. The narrative has been embedded into the culture of clinical practice at our organization, Massachusetts General Hospital (MGH), for many years. How that happened is a narrative itself, because it is the story of how an idea became reality, and it is a story we hope will be replicated in other institutions.

In this chapter, you read how to create an environment that is open to narratives and then review the strategies we used—and continue to use—at MGH to embed narratives into the culture of clinical practice. This chapter also provides direction on coaching, which is necessary not only for embedding narratives into the culture, but also for ensuring that narratives serve their intended purpose.

Embedding Narratives Into a Culture of Clinical Practice

To achieve a narrative culture, clinicians had to understand what narratives were and how they would be used; leaders had to become comfortable "unbundling" the narrative and in creating a narrative culture on their units; and narratives had to become visible within the organization. The strategies used at MGH to embed narratives into the culture are presented here.

Educational Sessions

In order for narratives to become embedded in the culture, it was important for clinicians and leadership to understand what narratives were—and, just as importantly, what they were not—and how they could be used to understand the knowledge embedded in clinical practice. Educational sessions were held centrally, at the unit level as well as on all shifts, including weekends. The sessions allowed for clinicians to ask questions, tell verbal narratives, and receive feedback. From these sessions, clinicians were able to begin to think of narratives as a way to describe their everyday practice rather than the earlier view of some that the narratives were highly edited dramatic stories. Clinicians were also given the opportunity for one-on-one consultation with experts who would work with them to help write their narratives.

Critical to the success of any initiative is the support of unit-based leadership, and this was true of creating a narrative culture. Although Nursing was familiar with clinical narratives because of its application by Dr. Patricia Benner (1984), members of the other disciplines—Occupational Therapy, Physical Therapy, Respiratory Therapy, Social Work, and Speech and Language Pathology—were not. Sessions were held with leadership to review narratives and practice unbundling them. It was important that leaders developed a level of comfort so that they could engage with clinicians to help them reflect on their practice and therefore develop their practice.

Publications

An organization makes visible and important what it values. This was true for embedding narratives into the work and thinking of clinicians at MGH. Every issue of *Caring Headlines*, the bimonthly Nursing and Patient Care Services newsletter, included a narrative written by a clinician. Following the narrative, the senior vice president for patient care and chief nurse writes a commentary that unbundles the narrative. The visibility of the narrative and the attention paid to it by executive leadership was a clear message that narratives were an essential and highly valued part of professional practice development in Nursing and Patient Care Services (NPCS).

Awards Programs

The use of clinical narratives to describe the clinician's practice in the care of patients and families led to their inclusion in the portfolios for award applications. In the application process for numerous NPCS awards, clinicians were able to reflect on the criteria for the award and then select a narrative in which the criteria were demonstrated in their practice. Often during the award ceremony, the recipient would be asked to read the narrative, and a member of leadership would then unbundle the narrative. Again, highlighting the narrative and unbundling it demonstrated the importance of the narrative.

The Clinical Recognition Program

The Clinical Recognition Program at MGH is based on the Dreyfus Model of Skill Acquisition (2004) and the work of Dr. Patricia Benner (1984). Dr. Benner used narratives to apply the Dreyfus Model to identify skill levels of nurses. Narratives allowed us to develop the themes and criteria in our first-of-its-kind interdisciplinary model (described in Chapter 1). Recognition at each level requires the clinician to write a narrative.

Annual Performance Reviews

Executive leadership at MGH set the expectation that annually each clinician would write a narrative to facilitate reflective practice. In order to operationalize this, leadership had to find a way that felt developmental and met and supported the clinicians where they were in their understanding and comfort in the narrative process.

At times the clinician's director would ask the clinician to relate a verbal narrative; as the clinician did, the director would take notes so that the clinician would have an outline for writing up the narrative. The expectation would be set that the following year, the narrative would be written prior to the evaluation. During the performance review, the director unbundles the narrative with the clinician. The dialogue which occurs around the narrative, in addition to the other components of the annual performance appraisal—manager's review, clinician's self-evaluation, and peer review—all inform the mutual development of professional development goals for the upcoming year.

Coaching the Clinical Narrative: The Role of Leadership

We hope that after reading the narratives and commentaries that you have recognized the opportunity this approach offers in uncovering and articulating the knowledge and skill embedded in clinical practice. The benefits we have discovered come from not only the writing of the narratives but also in leadership sitting with the clinician to continue the conversation on it. For many of the leaders, this time with the clinician has become a coaching opportunity. The ability to effectively coach their staff is a key leadership competency and yet one that may not be utilized enough.

In a 2011 *New Yorker* article, Atul Gawande, an author and surgeon, wrote that after clinicians reach competent practice, they do not receive individual, ongoing coaching in the way an athlete would. He wondered whether a coach would improve his surgical practice—it did. We believe that the use of narratives provides leaders an opportunity to coach their staff in reflecting on and developing their practice. While the coaching role is a key leadership competency, one hears from leaders that they do not spend enough time coaching staff, especially their competent or high performers. Gawande notes that in medicine, and we would add in nursing and the health professions, "expertise is thought to be not a static condition but one that doctors must build and sustain for themselves. Coaching in pro sports... holds that, no matter how well prepared people are in their formative years, few can achieve and maintain their best performance on their own."

We recognize that any search engine will spew thousands of articles, books, and tips on how to be an effective coach. It is not our intent to delve into the literature on this topic, and we instead state that for leaders to be effective coaches, they must be in partnership with their staff. Coaching is built on mutual trust. The individuals being coached must know that the coach will listen to them, process what is being said, reflect back to them through thoughtful questions, and give honest, constructive feedback.

Knowing what the individual needs to be effectively coached allows the leader to effectively coach. Consider the need for the coach to "listen." Directors at MGH create space and time for clinicians to share their narratives, following the formal performance appraisal session. A mutually agreed upon time is arranged in their office. Electronic devices are muted, and the focus is on the clinicians and their narrative. Directors will have the clinicians read their narrative aloud; this allows for further reflection by the clinicians as they return to the situation.

After hearing the story, the director begins the process of "unbundling" the narrative. By unbundling, we mean asking the clinicians to further describe and reflect on the narrative they just told. It is important to stay within the story at this point; larger lessons or situations similar to what has occurred can be discussed later. For now, focus on the story the clinician is telling you. As we have described earlier, knowledge is embedded in the practice and can become invisible or second nature to the clinician. The director's role is to allow the clinicians, through questions and curiosity, to reflect on their actions to make them visible to recognize opportunities for growth and change in situations that did not go well and the opportunity to recognize what they would do "next time."

When clinicians write their narratives, there are many forces at work. They could be doing it as part of an administrative exercise (i.e., as part of their performance appraisal), to be leveled as part of a recognition program, or to assist them and/or their colleagues in better understanding the dynamics of an interaction or patient illness. Whatever the reason, the clinicians are entrusting their stories to you. In the stories they might have succeeded or failed. The story could be as immediate as having happened that day or something that they have carried with them for years. They are allowing you to share in the intimacy of the care they provide their patients, the relationships they have with their colleagues, and their viewpoint on their professional work. When viewed from that light, the accountability and trust that is placed on leadership can be a heavy burden, but it's also a privilege.

Creating an Environment for Narratives

Leaders need to believe in the importance of the narrative in developing practice before they ever discuss implementation of this work on the unit. Clinicians have little time and patience for "busy work." If directors/managers come to the staff and tell them that they have to write a narrative because "administration" says they have to, then their efforts are bound to fail. Instead, leaders need to sit back and ask themselves several questions:

- Do you believe that clinicians' interactions with patients, families, and colleagues shape who they are and how they do their work?

- Do you believe that with experience clinicians are able to determine the most salient aspects of the patient's care and that this knowledge should be shared?

- Do you believe that clinicians' exposure to all facets of the human condition leaves them vulnerable and that there is a need to support them as they process these experiences?

If you answered yes to any of these questions, the narrative is a tool that may be helpful to you as you work with and develop the clinicians you manage. Now that you are willing to look at implementing the narrative on your unit, the question becomes, "How do I start?"

Creating a narrative culture means that you are creating an environment that values and supports the care of patients. You do this by talking about the work of clinicians caring for patients.

When you first begin talking about narratives, you will often hear clinicians say, "We do that already." That is true; we tell the stories of our work—over breaks, at change of shift, or outside of work. What is different with the clinical narrative is that the story is not just greeted with nods and agreement; it is followed with questions. Clinicians are asked to reflect on their work: What they did, why they did it, and what they wished they had done. This type of questioning does not usually occur during the informal discussions clinicians have.

Creating a narrative culture takes time and commitment, but it is based on the environment of practice and development. If that culture is present on your unit or department, moving to narratives will seem like a natural progression.

Getting Started

Putting pen to paper is a stressful experience for many clinicians. The fears range from worry about grammatical challenges to writer's block. Those fears often stand in the way of the clinician writing a narrative. It is important to think of this fear as a developmental step that the clinicians need to overcome as they advance in their profession. By doing this the director/manager can support the clinician with the same support he or she would use if the clinician was facing a fear in the clinical arena.

Many clinicians feel comfortable beginning this process by talking through their narrative. Sitting with the director, manager, or clinical specialist and simply discussing a patient or situation where the clinicians feel they made a difference, where something went well, or where systems broke down may feel less foreboding than having to write a narrative.

As the clinicians discuss their narrative, you may want to take a few notes about the story. By doing this you are cueing the clinicians into areas they may want to flesh out when they write their narrative or simply have them reflect on. Clinicians who casually say, "I knew something was wrong," have within them an area of embedded knowledge that should be delved into. Many times it is impossible for the clinicians to put into the narrative all they were thinking and experiencing at that moment; consequently, the director/manager must help tease out the story within the story through coaching. Following the discussion, the clinician is able, with the help of the notes that you provided and your discussion, to write the narrative.

THE NARRATIVE LIVES ON

Many times you will be asked, "Why do narratives have to be written?" Writing has gone out of fashion for many people, and so, as was mentioned earlier, putting pen to paper or fingers to keyboard is daunting. But the experience of writing allows for a thoughtfulness that is lacking when an issue is discussed. Each word and phrase is formed and evaluated and lives on long after our voices are silenced.

Summary

In 1996, the decision of the senior vice president for patient care and chief nurse to focus attention and resources to embedding narratives into the culture of NPCS was not without controversy, but as the preceding chapters have shown, that decision has benefited clinicians, their colleagues, and most importantly, patients and their families. Using narratives to fully understand the four levels of practice across the disciplines allowed us to create our Clinical Recognition Program. The inclusion of narratives as an annual part of the clinicians' performance appraisal has allowed for a meaningful exchange between leadership and clinicians about their practice and their goals. The inclusion of narratives in applicant award portfolios allowed award criteria to come alive.

There are many reasons for the commitment to excellence in NPCS: transformative leadership, an expert and caring staff, an organizational culture focused on excellence. But we also believe that creating an opportunity for clinicians to reflect on their practice through the use of the narrative assisted us in our journey.

References

Benner, P. (1984). *From novice to expert: Excellence and power in clinical nursing practice.* Menlo Park, CA: Addison-Wesley.

Dreyfus, S. E. (2004). The five stage model of adult skill acquisition. *Bulletin of Science, Technology & Society, 24*(3), 177–181.

Gawande, A. (2011). Personal best. *The New Yorker,* October, 44–53.

Appendix A
Describing Practice Through Clinical Narratives: Guidelines for Clinicians

Your clinical narrative should be a first-person "story" about a clinical event or situation that holds some special meaning for you. Your narrative should be an honest reflection of your current clinical practice.

Choosing a Topic for Your Narrative

Your narrative can be based on one or more of the following:

- A situation in which you feel your intervention really made a difference in the patient's outcome—for example, you recognized a change in the patient's condition or an opportunity to intervene.

- A situation that you commonly confront in your practice—for example, ethical concerns or a rapidly changing clinical situation.

- A situation that was particularly demanding—for example, caring for a dying patient or a situation of conflict.

- A situation that you think captures the essence of your discipline—for example, when you leave work and say, "I was at my best today. I made a difference."

Writing Your Clinical Narrative

In writing a clinical narrative, you should include the following:

- ❏ Information about yourself, such as your name, title, unit, and length of time in practice

- ❏ The context of the clinical situation: where it took place, time of day, shift, existing conditions

- ❏ A detailed description of what happened

- ❏ Why this clinical situation is important to you

- ❏ What your concerns were at the time

- ❏ What you were thinking about as the situation was taking place

- ❏ What you were feeling during and after the situation

- ❏ What, if anything, you found most demanding

- ❏ Important conversations you had with the patient, family, and members of the healthcare team or other relevant parties

The following tips will help you write your narrative:

- ❏ Present your story as a first-person account.

- ❏ Change the patient's name and any other identifying information in order to protect confidentiality.

- ❏ "Tell" your story into a tape recorder and then transcribe the tape and edit it, tightening it and filling in any needed details.

- ❏ Tell the complete story first and then edit it to include the essential details.

Editing Your Clinical Narrative

After you've written your initial narrative, it's important to take the time to edit it:

❏ Review your story with a colleague who has also cared for the patient. This may help you capture the description you want.

❏ Have someone read your narrative who doesn't know the patient to see if there are questions or if you missed information. An outside reader can help you fill in familiar information you may have taken for granted.

❏ When you edit your narrative, avoid vague summary statements or general phrases that do not communicate what actually occurred. Examples include:

   ❏ "I analyzed the possible dangers to the patient and took action."

   ❏ "I gave emotional support."

   ❏ "The patient's improving."

❏ More specific ways of stating what occurred include:

   ❏ "The blood pressure was dropping and the pulse rate was rising; I sensed the patient was going into shock. I immediately called the intern."

   ❏ "I sat and talked with the patient about how to tell his family about the diagnosis."

   ❏ "The patient is able to sit independently, transfer out of bed with assistance, and is progressing with gait activities on the parallel bars and with a walker."

❏ Be sure you have included your concerns or what you were anticipating when you took a particular action; this gives a window into your judgment. For example, "I thought the patient would be resistant, so I decided to...."

As we end this chapter and the book, we hope you are intrigued and excited about the opportunities narratives can bring to you, your unit/department, and your organization. But we recognize that you might also harbor some doubts. At MGH, when we want to know if an organizational initiative is working, we ask a group that has no trouble telling us the truth—we ask our staff. Here is what they told us about writing and sharing narratives:

- I was completely against having to write an annual narrative. Now I find I am upset if my director does not spend time discussing it with me.

- I made a medication error, and I felt so terrible. And then a nurse I really respect read his narrative about an error he made. I realized, if someone like him can make an error and learn from it and then share it, then I could too.

- I remembered a narrative another nurse shared on a patient who was going into septic shock, so when my patient began to get into trouble, I thought, "This is it. This is septic shock." I had studied it in school, of course, but her narrative stayed with me and allowed me to consider septic shock sooner than I would have.

- I really struggled coming up with a narrative. Nothing seemed important and special enough. I was complaining to my friend, whom I work with, and he said what about the patient you cared for that you got out of restraints? I didn't think it was anything, but I was desperate so I wrote a paragraph and met with my nursing director. It was only in talking with her about it that I realized all I did and how the rest of the staff bought into my plan because they trusted me. I really didn't know all that went into what I had done.

Appendix B
The Levels of Practice

Clinicians in Nursing and Patient Care Services (NPCS) at Massachusetts General Hospital have long valued their role in caring for patients and families. The Clinical Recognition Program provides a way to formally recognize professional clinical staff for their expertise. The program recognizes that valuable contributions are made by staff at every level, and excellence is a goal common to all.

The levels and criteria that follow were developed through analyzing the narratives of clinicians in the six disciplines in NPCS—Nursing, Occupational Therapy, Physical Therapy, Respiratory Therapy, Social Work, and Speech–Language Pathology—through interviews and through validating the criteria with clinicians and leadership.

TABLE B.1 Levels of Practice: Nursing—The Clinician–Patient Relationship

ENTRY	CLINICIAN	ADVANCED CLINICIAN	CLINICAL SCHOLAR
Demonstrates care and concern for patients and families.	Individualizes care based upon the knowledge of the patient and the family.	Modifies interventions based on a deep understanding of patient and family needs attained through past experiences.	Intuitively uses self in the therapeutic relationship as a means to enhance care.
Recognizes how the clinician–patient relationship affects the patient experience.	Recognizes needs and advocates for patient based on knowledge of condition.	Advocacy for the patient causes the clinician to challenge systems and practices; tries to identify patterns in systems or processes of care that impact patient and families.	Actively empowers and advocates for patients and families to maximize their participation in decision-making and goal setting.
Begins to recognize the differences in how patients and families react to illness and treatment.	Has awareness of own values and how they affect interactions and relationships.	Is open and inclusive of others' values.	Respects others' values and suspends judgment.
	Recognizes that cultural differences need to be considered in developing clinician–patient relationships. Focus is on identifying cultural norms.	Alters interpersonal exchanges to meet cultural differences.	Plans constructive interventions based on patient's values.
		Develops and values collaborative relationships with patients and families.	Demonstrates scope of responsibility and accountability for clinical practice.
			Effectively elicits cultural beliefs and values from patients and integrates these into overall patient management.
			Challenges and shapes systems on the unit and hospitalwide to achieve best possible outcomes.

© Massachusetts General Hospital

TABLE B.2 Levels of Practice: Nursing—Clinical Knowledge and Decision-Making

ENTRY	CLINICIAN	ADVANCED CLINICIAN	CLINICAL SCHOLAR
Safely implements nursing interventions and procedures in the care of the patient.	Demonstrates mastery of technical skills.	Acts as a resource to colleagues in relation to a particular patient population.	Is recognized as an expert in area of interest and/or specialization.
Organizes and prioritizes care, with assistance as necessary.	Through the ongoing experience of caring for patients and families, recognizes patterns that refine and influence future practice.	Past experience allows clinician to focus on "probabilities versus possibilities" when assessing and caring for patients.	Understands the impact of illness on the lives of patient and family.
Begins to integrate theoretical knowledge with the practical experience of caring for patients.	Is adaptable and flexible in managing clinical situations.	Demonstrates a spirit of inquiry as it relates to clinical practice; wants to know why.	Demonstrates exquisite foresight in anticipating and planning to meet patient and family problems and concerns.
Understands unit operations that support the delivery of patient care.	Begins to take clinically sound risks.	Initiates independent learning based on her/his needs.	Applies and shares relevant research with colleagues.
	Seeks out and utilizes resources and colleagues to validate information in order to maintain the standards of care and practice.	Is adaptable and flexible in managing unexpected clinical situations.	Critically evaluates own decision-making and judgments.
	Recognizes the challenges of, and develops strategies for, prioritizing and organizing care.	Feels increasingly comfortable in taking clinically sound risks.	Consistently takes clinically sound risks.
	Recognizes the responsibility and accountability for her/his own practice.	Views clinical decision-making holistically, including both prior experiences and current clinical situation.	Independently seeks out opportunities to learn, teach, and influence.
			Successfully organizes and coordinates multiple activities, requests and needs.
			Implements innovative approaches to meet the needs of patients and families.

© Massachusetts General Hospital

TABLE B.3   Levels of Practice: Nursing—Teamwork and Collaboration

ENTRY	CLINICIAN	ADVANCED CLINICIAN	CLINICAL SCHOLAR
Understands the role of other disciplines in the care of patients.	Seeks and values collegial relationships between nursing and other disciplines.	Acts as a resource to colleagues or refers colleagues to others as necessary.	Skillfully negotiates conflict to promote collaboration.
Identifies the resources that are available for patients and families.	Provides guidance to less-experienced staff (i.e., precepts).	Anticipates patient/family needs and is proactive in initiating consults and/or engaging other team members.	Peer development focuses on elevating the standard of practice as a whole. Implements unique and innovative approaches to meeting patient, family, unit, and practice concerns.
Utilizes the assistance of resources and colleagues.	Contributes to the effective operation of her/his unit.	Promotes the development of collaborative relationships with colleagues and peers by communicating in a constructive manner.	Aware of and supports unit's and colleagues' needs through supportive and non-judgmental behaviors.
Understands unit-based structures that enhance communication between team members.	Understands her/his role as a member of the healthcare team. Participates in interdisciplinary forums that promote an integrated approach to patient care.		Leads/coordinates activities that affect the quality of care on the unit and/or patient population. Achieves credibility. Peers and members of the health-care team seek clinician's consultation. Works effectively on hospitalwide teams and initiatives.

© Massachusetts General Hospital

TABLE B.4 Levels of Practice: Physical Therapy and Occupational Therapy—The Clinician–Patient Relationship

ENTRY	CLINICIAN	ADVANCED CLINICIAN	CLINICAL SCHOLAR
Rapport and communication			
Is aware of own values and recognizes how one's own values affect interactions and relationships.	Is open to others' values.	Respects others' values.	Respects others' values and suspends judgment.
Demonstrates comfort in establishing and maintaining rapport with patients.	Is able to interact effectively with variety of patients/families, modifying own communication style as needed.	Increasingly aware of complex patient/family dynamics and actively seeks to validate perceptions for purpose of factoring them into clinical impression.	Intuitively uses self in the therapeutic relationship as a means to enhance care.
Beginning to perceive subtleties in patient/family dynamics and incorporates this insight into interactions with both.	Increasingly aware of complex patient/family dynamics and impact on clinical impression.	Recognizes importance of patient assuming responsibility for portions of own care and makes this a key component of intervention strategy.	Effectively adjusts approach to patient/family communication, thereby maximizing rapport and facilitating open exchange of information.
Provides accurate information/input regarding a patient's PT or OT needs to the healthcare team.	Recognizes importance of patient assuming responsibility for portions of own care.		Empowers patients and family to take control of their well-being; employs focused patient/family education to that end.

continues

TABLE B.4 *continued*

ENTRY	CLINICIAN	ADVANCED CLINICIAN	CLINICAL SCHOLAR
Interface with clinical decision-making			
Considers knowledge of patient and family when implementing standards of care.	Effectively gathers pertinent, subjective data from patient/family to make clinical decisions.	Efficiently gathers pertinent, subjective data from patient/family to make clinical decisions. Clusters information to understand patient life roles, functional needs. This data drives examination, evaluation, and intervention.	Listens carefully to patients and uses them as a primary source of data. Negotiates realistic goals and intervention plan based on patient's values.
Advocacy			
Recognizes need for advocacy and brings individual patient needs to the interdisciplinary team.	Recognizes common advocacy issues across patients.	Recognizes common advocacy issues across patients and seeks assistance to organize and plan approach to achieve advocacy goals beyond the individual patient. Consistently voices and supports professional opinion even if it differs from other interdisciplinary team members.	Sees advocacy as a key professional role of the PT/OT. Confidently approaches MD, other health professionals, third-party payers, etc. to advocate for patient's needs. Uses knowledge gained with patients to advocate for issues of health/public policy. Consistently identifies patient and systemic needs across disciplines and advocates beyond discipline-specific issues.

ENTRY	CLINICIAN	ADVANCED CLINICIAN	CLINICAL SCHOLAR
Cultural competence			
Recognizes that cultural differences need to be considered in developing clinician–patient relationships. Focus is on identifying cultural norms.	Identifies a variety of cultural factors that may affect treatment goals and outcomes.	Understands factors that affect developing rapport with patients of various cultural backgrounds and considers those factors in developing treatment plan and projecting outcomes.	Effectively elicits cultural beliefs and values from patients and integrates these into overall patient management.

TABLE B.5 Levels of Practice: Physical Therapy and Occupational Therapy—Clinical Decision-Making

ENTRY	CLINICIAN	ADVANCED CLINICIAN	CLINICAL SCHOLAR
Self-assessment			
Developing accuracy in self-assessment within a limited scope of practice (e.g., diagnosis-specific).	Recognizes limitations in knowledge and skills. Employs active experimentation as a learning mode and reflection on results directs development of treatment skills.	Accurately self-assesses across a range and complexity of diagnoses. Recognizes limitations in knowledge and skills, and developmental needs for gaining expertise in a more specialized aspect of care. Reflects on results of active experimentation issued as a method to develop treatment skills and achieve outcomes. Able to identify own developmental needs for gaining expertise in a more specialist aspect of care. Analyzes clinical decision-making and identifies multiple sources of error.	Continually critically evaluates own decision-making and judgments. Accurately identifies boundaries of knowledge and skill and efficiently confers with referral source regarding patient needs. Demonstrates exquisite foresight in anticipating own developmental needs, often developing skills outside PT area of specialization.

ENTRY	CLINICIAN	ADVANCED CLINICIAN	CLINICAL SCHOLAR
Clinical reasoning			
Knowledge, Examination, Evaluation/dx, Prognosis, Intervention, Exercise prescription			
Knowledge tends to be compartmentalized into diagnostic categories.	Demonstrates a solid knowledge base and framework for practice across a range of patient complexity. Sees diagnosis as a framework to initiate decisions about examination.	Understands the range of variability within diagnosis and integrates data that does not "fit" into clinical decision-making.	Patient's medical diagnosis serves to establish context in which examination data are gathered and evaluated, but it does not drive the decision-making process per se.
Assessments reflect more short-range predictions versus view of patient at end of episode of care.			
Developing skills in prioritization of patient assessment/examination procedures.	Assessments reflect the ability to integrate pathophysiology, co-morbidities and psychosocial issues.	Clinician confidently and efficiently predicts outcomes beyond a single episode of care and considers the long-term needs of the patient.	Accurately and efficiently clusters findings from multiple data sources and identifies meaningful patterns based on prior experience.
Utilizes other staff as primary source of knowledge and to assist with clinical interpretation of new information.	Clinical impression is made within the context of individual needs and goals.	Takes initiative to identify learning needs and resources. Follows through and shares information with peers in a timely manner.	Patient care is outcome driven, with outcomes defined in terms of goals that have been established in conjunction with the patient and his/her identified needs.
	Clinician begins to predict outcomes across an episode of care.		
Identifies relationship between impairments and function, but may tend to view functional training as an end in itself versus one way to achieve impairment resolution.	Takes initiative to identify learning needs and resources.	Transfers skills and knowledge confidently into unfamiliar situations and efficiently identifies new learning needs.	Selectively designs and implements an exercise program that focuses on most critical issues to be addressed.
	Transfers skills and knowledge to a variety of patient care situations.	Efficiently identifies and plans for patients' needs, including patients who will not benefit from PT/OT.	

continues

TABLE B.5 *continued*

Clinical reasoning *continued*

Knowledge, Examination, Evaluation/dx, Prognosis, Intervention, Exercise prescription

ENTRY	CLINICIAN	ADVANCED CLINICIAN	CLINICAL SCHOLAR
Demonstrates beginning skills in weighing impact of co-morbidities/anticipated disease progression.	Efficiently identifies and plans for patients' needs.	Anticipates individual variation in patient response and has a variety of options and resources to meet patient needs.	Recognizes the relative relevance of data from many sources and relies on minimum data set necessary to form decisions.
Recognizes scope of intervention strategies to include direct, compensatory, and consultation. Primarily uses direct intervention methods.	Sees key impairments as related to functional problems and prioritizes goals and treatments accordingly.	Efficiently clusters information from a variety of sources. More selective and efficient utilization of manual techniques, along with other methods of intervention to maximize outcomes given increased managed care pressures.	Recognizes when further tests and measures will not add value to the clinical decision-making process. Identifies when findings do not fit together and one's PT or OT tools cannot validate the suspected cause of patient's problem. Confidently approaches MD or other health professionals to advocate for patient's needs.
Consistently plans for patient needs, able to recognize when plan needs revision. Modification of plan is more likely the result of a reflective process than an automatic one.	Utilizes varied manual techniques along with other methods of intervention to achieve outcomes. Continually progresses patient-based, ongoing reassessment.	Demonstrates clinically sound risk-taking.	Highly selective and efficient in the use of manual techniques in combination with other methods of intervention to achieve predicted outcomes given managed care pressures.
Provides broad-based treatment approach that includes all patient-identified problems that relate to functional limitations.	Treatment approach reflects prioritized problems. Seeks guidance to integrate specific pathophysiology and surgical intervention into the development of exercise programs.	Treatment approach is selective and prioritizes problems. Selectively utilizes functional activities to achieve desired outcomes. Specifically integrates pathophysiology and surgical intervention into development of exercise programs.	Demonstrates thorough and consistent foresight in anticipating patients' developmental needs.

ENTRY	CLINICIAN	ADVANCED CLINICIAN	CLINICAL SCHOLAR
Evidence-based practice			
Recognizes research as the basis of practice. Seeks broad-based information, which is diagnosis-driven.	Utilizes resources and seeks appropriate assistance to validate research information for sound, clinical decision-making.	Through the readings of scientific literature is able to identify current issues and trends in practice. Evidence drawn from the literature is actively pursued to support clinical practice. Incorporates research findings into clinical practice.	Articulates theoretical foundation for practice and uses available evidence from a variety of sources to inform clinical decision-making. Identifies gaps in the available evidence base for practice and helps to bring into focus the research questions critical to moving practice forward.
Accountability and responsibility			
Recognizes the responsibility and accountability for his/her own clinical practice in relationship to the immediate needs of the patient. Sees lack of patient progress as immediately implicating own skills and abilities as less than adequate. Recognizes the need to prioritize and organize care.	Assumes responsibility for communicating with and educating other team members, as needed, to facilitate integration of patient's PT and OT needs into current plan of care (including d/c plan).	Has learned to share responsibility for care with patient and is able to let go of need to "make every patient better." Life experience and knowledge gained outside of the professional work environment adds to the skill in managing patient-care needs. Demonstrates involvement in activities that contribute to the improvement of the unit/department/profession.	Experiences a sense of accountability for patient progress toward goals. If not progressing as anticipated asks self "What have I not figured out?" Demonstrates leadership in activities that contribute to the advancement of the unit/department/profession. Demonstrates exquisite foresight in anticipating and pursuing patient's developing needs across entire episode of care.

continues

TABLE B.5 *continued*

ENTRY	CLINICIAN	ADVANCED CLINICIAN	CLINICAL SCHOLAR
Education/consultation			
Patient and family education			
Consistently incorporates patient/family education into treatment plans.	Adapts patient/family education plan based on individual needs.	Efficiently adapts patient/family education plan based on individual needs.	In consultation with the patient, develops a specific education plan that allows patient to have maximal control.
Participates in community education.	Participates/assists in the planning of community education.		Educates PTs/OTs and other disciplines beyond the facility via publications/presentations.
Student education			
Participates in clinical education program with observational/part-time clinical experiences.	Participates in clinical education program with entry-level students and interns.	Participates in clinical education program with all levels of students. Works with individuals that are involved in transitional degree and residency programs.	Works efficiently and effectively with all students/staff on educational and professional development issues.
Demonstrates basic knowledge of the teaching-learning process.	Develops clear objectives and plans student learning activities. Provides feedback of student performance.	In conjunction with the student, individualizes goals/learning activities. Evaluates student performance against clear standards and communicates strengths/developmental needs to participants.	Efficiently/effectively identifies student/staff learning needs and knowledge gaps. Assists in development of learning goals/plans to facilitate development of clinical skills.

ENTRY	CLINICIAN	ADVANCED CLINICIAN	CLINICAL SCHOLAR
Consultation			
Educates team about professional role.	Consults with other healthcare team members regarding patient needs for services.	Consults with less-experienced staff and peers to maximize patient outcomes.	Achieves credibility; consultation is sought by peers and members of the healthcare team in planning patient care. Identifies and utilizes appropriate resources to provide outcome-focused consultation. Recognizes common characteristics within specific diagnostic groups and is effective in influencing the development of disease-specific management (e.g., pathway development).

© Massachusetts General Hospital

TABLE B.6 Levels of Practice: Physical Therapy and Occupational Therapy—Teamwork and Collaboration

ENTRY	CLINICIAN	ADVANCED CLINICIAN	CLINICAL SCHOLAR
Interdisciplinary team			
Demonstrates comfort in role as a team member and is developing awareness of professional boundaries.	Educates team members, as needed, to facilitate integration of patient's PT and OT needs into plan of care.	Instills confidence in colleagues.	Effective in alerting team to needs of patient that may extend beyond scope of one's clinical practice.
Seeks and values collaborative relationships with other disciplines to enhance patient management.		Recognizes the need for consultation and institutes referrals that will result in mobilization of resources to meet patient and family needs.	Skillfully negotiates conflict to promote collaboration.
Developing skills in negotiation/managing conflicts in roles.		Consistently demonstrates the flexibility and ability to accommodate the needs of the service and the patient on a daily basis.	Implements unique and innovative approaches to meeting developmental needs of self and others.
Peer development focuses on learning needs of individual peers.			Views team education as a central part of role and integrates it into daily routines.
Support personnel			
Utilizes a variety of support staff to assist with achievement of patient goals.	Assimilates pertinent data, communicates to selected team members, and delegates appropriately to achieve desired outcomes.	Efficiently assimilates pertinent data, communicates to selected team members, and delegates appropriately to achieve desired outcomes and maximize ability to manage entire caseload.	Clearly defines own role and that of various support personnel and is able to accurately and efficiently match a patient's needs to appropriate support resources to achieve optimal outcomes.

ENTRY	CLINICIAN	ADVANCED CLINICIAN	CLINICAL SCHOLAR
System			
Contributes to the effective operation of the department. Identifies the value of operations-improvement activities.	Identifies problems related to practice and/or systems.	Identifies systems or practice issues and potential solutions as part of professional role. Actively participates in operations-improvement activities.	Challenges and shapes the system to maximize the benefits for patient care. Peer development focuses on elevating the standard of practice as a whole. Leads/coordinates operations-improvement activities affecting his/her work area and/or patient population.

TABLE B.7 Levels of Practice: Physical Therapy and Occupational Therapy—Movement

ENTRY	CLINICIAN	ADVANCED CLINICIAN	CLINICAL SCHOLAR
Motor coordination and skill			
Palpate, Facilitate versus inhibit movement			
Developing skills in being able to facilitate desired movement pattern while assisting patients with functional activities. Developing skills of palpation as tools of clinical practice.	Skills of palpation, observation, and guidance play an important role in decision-making and are effectively incorporated into clinical practice. Selects hands-on techniques for the purpose of examination and/or achieving desired patient outcomes.	Efficiently selects and adapts skills of palpation, observation, and guidance based on previous experience.	Employs highly refined skills of palpation, observation, and guidance of movement as tools of clinical practice. Uses hands-on techniques selectively and in a manner that supports rather than detracts from the primary focus, that of understanding the patient's problem.
Analyze movement and respond			
Judgment, Planned versus automatic responses			
Developing skill in analyzing movement and identifying normal versus abnormal movement patterns. Effectively plans for and applies hands-on techniques. Recognizes need to modify planned intervention, but specific action may require reflective rather than automatic process.	Demonstrates skill in identifying key components of movement related to impaired functional performance. Seeks guidance for complex patients.	Anticipates key components of movement related to improving functional performance. Demonstrates ability to automatically adjust hand placements to achieve desired patient response.	Analysis of movement is used as a guide to patient care (i.e., linking the movement that is observed or felt to an intrinsic sense of what is "normal" and determining how it relates to the patient's ability to function). Is able to finely adjust hands-on techniques to meet the needs of individual patient-care situations.

© Massachusetts General Hospital

TABLE B.8 Levels of Practice: Respiratory Therapy—Movement

ENTRY	CLINICIAN	ADVANCED CLINICIAN	CLINICAL SCHOLAR
Demonstrates care and concern for patients and families.	Able to effectively communicate with patients/families regarding specifics of the respiratory care provided.	Adjusts therapy based on needs and concerns of patient and family.	Anticipates patient's/family's needs and offers assistance to patient/family to enhance care.
Recognizes patients' needs and advocates for patients.	Individualizes care based upon the knowledge of the patient and the family.	Encourages patient/families to participate in patient's care.	Develops creative approaches to encourage patient/family participation.
Recognizes the need to communicate with patients/families regarding specifics of respiratory care.	Recognizes that cultural differences need to be considered.	Adjusts care plan to provide culturally sensitive care.	Provides emotional and informational support to patients and families and modifies subsequent discussion based on where the patient and the family are with regard to the stages of coping and acceptance.
Treats all patients with the same level of respect and professionalism.	Selects relevant information to share differently among patients, caregivers, and professionals and assures their understanding.	Is open and inclusive of others' values.	
		Uses past experiences to adjust treatment.	Separates personal feelings from moral and ethical dilemmas.
		Anticipates patient's needs and sets priorities.	Respects values and suspends judgment.
			Challenges systems to provide the best patient outcomes.

TABLE B.9 Levels of Practice: Respiratory Therapy—Clinical Knowledge

ENTRY	CLINICIAN	ADVANCED CLINICIAN	CLINICAL SCHOLAR
Understands the need to incorporate clinical competencies into the delivery of care.	Understands clinical and lab data and utilizes the information to appropriately provide patient care.	Serves as a consultant for clinical competencies.	Serves as department resource for developing clinical competencies.
Capable of performing routine technical aspects of respiratory care.	Able to effectively incorporate clinical competencies into the delivery of care.	Has mastered technical aspects of respiratory care.	Clinical and technical expert in area of specialization.
Provides acceptable documentation.	Appropriately documents rationale for therapy.	Effectively documents goals of therapy.	Uses documentation to effectively integrate patient care plan.
Recognizes the need to incorporate clinical and laboratory data into the assessment of patients.	Technically competent.	Is familiar with relevant research findings.	Applies relevant research findings to clinical practice.
Attends rounds when appropriate.	Actively participates in rounds.	Provides inservice education.	Recognizes the need for and develops continuing education programs.
Recognizes limits; utilizes resources appropriately.	Demonstrates clinically sound risk-taking.	Effective in influencing change for more appropriate respiratory care.	Develops innovative approaches to care.
Attends inservices.	Appropriately challenges physicians' orders.	Initiates independent learning based on his/her needs.	
Needs help setting priorities.	Actively participates in inservices.	Anticipates patient needs and sets priorities appropriately.	
Approach to patient care is rule-driven.	Draws conclusions on past experiences.		
	Matches rules with reality.		

TABLE B.10 Levels of Practice: Respiratory Therapy—Teamwork and Collaboration

ENTRY	CLINICIAN	ADVANCED CLINICIAN	CLINICAL SCHOLAR
Recognizes the need for a team approach to patient care.	Collaborates with members of the patient care team to develop an integrated care plan.	Actively seeks other health-care team members to provide an integrated care plan.	Leads and coordinates operation-improvement activities for clinical practice and system improvements.
Begins developing relationships with the healthcare team.	Identifies the need for improvement in the respiratory care department.	Develops solutions for implementing improvements in practice.	Consultation is sought by peers and other members of the healthcare team.
Benefits more from than contributes to teamwork.	Begins to see positive effect of own contribution to teamwork.	Mobilizes teamwork, contributes to more than benefits from teamwork.	Projects a professional image and positively influences practice for better patient care.
			Often leads teams.

© Massachusetts General Hospital

TABLE B.11 Levels of Practice: Social Work—The Clinician–Patient Relationship

ENTRY	CLINICIAN	ADVANCED CLINICIAN	CLINICAL SCHOLAR
Able to demonstrate empathic understanding of patients/families.	Able to be present; stay with, sit, and listen to patient's story and underlying effect; bearing witness to patient's story.	Capacity to use the self to enable effective working relationship.	Innovatively and creatively engages patients and families.
Ability to engage with diverse patient population (differing personalities, illnesses, social, economic, and cultural factors).	Able to sit with and respond to strong effect.	Capacity to work skillfully with a designated population of patients considering a multiplicity of factors (biological, psychological, social, cultural, and environmental).	Purposefully integrates transference/counter-transference to further the therapeutic alliance.
Ability to identify own personal reactions and seek appropriate support and supervision.	Capacity to work within the therapeutic relationship to develop mutually agreed upon goals with the patient.	Ability to enable patients to develop self-reliance, self-knowledge, and self-awareness to become empowered in their own treatment and care.	Establishes working relationships with help-resistant, difficult, complicated, multiproblem patients and families.
Learning to manage the professional relationships.	Capacity to encourage patients in self-reliance, maintaining a reasonable expectation of growth and change.	Ability to step back and objectively perceive the patient, the self, and the dynamics of interaction.	Integrates theoretical knowledge, clinical skills, and active and purposeful use of the self to guide the therapeutic intervention with patients and families.
	Ability to identify need for and to set appropriate boundaries with diverse patient populations.		

© Massachusetts General Hospital

TABLE B.12 Levels of Practice: Social Work—Clinical Knowledge and Decision-Making

ENTRY	CLINICIAN	ADVANCED CLINICIAN	CLINICAL SCHOLAR
Ability to gather psychosocial information from a variety of sources and use a broad theoretical framework to make an assessment.	Ability to simultaneously process patient/family information and social work theory.	Demonstrates working knowledge of multiple theories relevant to practice.	Demonstrates expertise in theory relevant to social work practice.
Able to employ relevant interventions based on assessment.	Ability to perform biopsychosocial assessments integrating theory and setting appropriate treatment plans (biopsychosocial, cultural, etc.).	Demonstrates expertise in diagnosis and clinical interventions.	Demonstrates ability to confidently, competently, and creatively treat patients and families using a variety of modalities.
Able to provide patient and family education regarding community and hospital resources.	Ability to intervene with patients and families using more than one treatment modality.	Demonstrates clinically sound risk-taking.	Ability to focus and prioritize treatment interventions in complex, multiproblem patient situations.
Seeks appropriate supervision and consultation.	Ability to recognize need for and provide psycho-education to patients and families.	Ability to discern/prioritize those patients and families that can benefit from clinical interventions.	Sought out to teach, supervise, and provide consultation to colleagues in own and other disciplines.
Appropriately uses protocols for clinical decision-making.	Demonstrates confidence and competence in familiar situations.	Incorporates in-depth patient and family education in area of own expertise.	Demonstrates wisdom in decision-making based on theoretical, clinical, and experiential knowledge.
	Ability to transfer skills and knowledge into unfamiliar situations.	Demonstrates confidence and competence in unfamiliar situations.	Demonstrates professional contributions to clinical knowledge and practice.
	Ability to prioritize based on patients' need.	Ability to teach/supervise colleagues.	
	Ability to mentor colleagues.	Ability to refer to and/or seek consultation from other appropriate healthcare providers.	

© Massachusetts General Hospital

TABLE B.13 Levels of Practice: Social Work—Teamwork and Collaboration

ENTRY	CLINICIAN	ADVANCED CLINICIAN	CLINICAL SCHOLAR
Identifies problems and seeks consultation.	Actively shares clinical knowledge (obtained from many sources) and own clinical impressions to keep others informed in order to provide quality, team-oriented patient care.	Incorporates multidisciplinary perspective in promoting quality, team-oriented patient care.	Able to effectively mobilize the interdisciplinary team to provide quality patient care.
Team membership characterized by thoughtful observation and information-sharing.		Able to articulate a point of view on the team that enables the team to comprehensively problem-solve.	Uses knowledge of the organization to identify and solve system and patient problems.
Works collaboratively and problem-solves with individual team members.	Able to articulate the social work perspective to promote problem-solving.	Assumes leadership in departmental Collaborative Leadership Teams.	Articulates the clinical expertise of social work on the team.
Joins actively in the work of the Collaborative Leadership Team.	Actively shares responsibility for getting the work of the Collaborative Leadership Team done.	Understands roles of other disciplines and is able to articulate the limitations of social work.	Sought for clinical expertise (consultation and referral).
	Provides support to social work and multidisciplinary colleagues.	Sought out by colleagues for consultation and referral.	Promotes team building in all its diversity.
	Understands the roles of other disciplines.	Provides consultation to interdisciplinary colleagues regarding psychosocial issues and patient/family behavior.	Promotes creativity and growth of peers.
	Attracts referrals and is sought out by colleagues for collaboration.	Chairs committees and task forces focused on patient care.	Chairs interdisciplinary committees and task forces focused on patient care.
		Utilizes conflict resolution skills in response to difficult situations and conflicts with colleagues.	

TABLE B.14 Levels of Practice: Speech–Language Pathology—The Clinician–Patient Relationship

ENTRY	CLINICIAN	ADVANCED CLINICIAN	CLINICAL SCHOLAR
Considers knowledge of patient and family when implementing standards of care.	Individualizes care based upon knowledge of patient and family attained through the therapeutic relationship.	Identifies and incorporates patient and family's best mode of learning.	Intuitively uses self in the therapeutic relationship as a means to enhance care.
Recognizes needs and advocates for patient based on knowledge of condition. May be disease driven.	Advocates based on individual patient and family needs.	Captures a patient's readiness to learn and responds accordingly.	Actively mobilizes and empowers patients and families.
Has self-awareness of one's own values and how one's own values affect interactions and relationships.	Is open to other's values.	Provides informational materials and emotional support to patients and families.	Respects values and suspends judgment.
Recognizes the uniqueness of each patient and their families and acknowledges cultural differences.	Selects relevant information to share differently among patients, caregivers, and professionals and assures their understanding.	Alters interpersonal exchanges to meet cultural differences.	Plans constructive interventions based on patient's values.
Understands the role of the patient and their family in developing realistic goals and expectations based on patient's needs and circumstances.	Provides informational materials and support to patients and families.	Shares relevant information with caregivers, professionals, patients, and family members. Subsequent discussion may be altered based on verbal and nonverbal responses to the information presented.	Works to build and maintain a relationship with patient and family that encourage self-reliance and independence.
Provides informational materials to patients and families.	Identifies patient's readiness to learn and evaluates patient's response to educational exchange.	Advocates for individuals and families and tries to identify institutional trends that require higher-level advocacy.	Advocates for patients at various levels: individual, institutional, state, and federal.
	Advocates for individual patients and families and utilizes knowledge of institutional patterns during advocacy.		Provides emotional and informational support to patients and families and modifies subsequent discussion based on where the patient and the family are with regard to the stages of coping and acceptance.

TABLE B.15 Levels of Practice: Speech–Language Pathology—Clinical Knowledge and Decision-Making

ENTRY	CLINICIAN	ADVANCED CLINICIAN	CLINICAL SCHOLAR
Utilizes resources and validates information to maintain standards of care and practice.	Demonstrates a solid knowledge base.	Anticipates needs and sets priorities.	Is recognized as an expert in an area of interest and/or specialization.
Recognizes the need to prioritize and organize care.	Demonstrates a mastery of skills.	Demonstrates spirit of inquiry as it relates to clinical practice.	Understands the meaning of illness to patient and family.
Recognizes research as the basis of clinical practice.	Initiates independent learning based on his/her needs.	Considers individual differences in normal and disordered communication and swallowing functions across the age span, as well as the role of sociocultural differences relevant to these functions.	Synthesizes knowledge and experience in anticipating and planning to meet patient and family needs.
Recognizes the responsibility and accountability for his/her own clinical practice.	Demonstrates clinically sound risk-taking.	Integrates relationships among medical diagnosis, symptoms, and reason for referral.	Applies relevant research findings to practice.
Utilizes a conscious, deliberate process to attain clinical decisions.	Is guided by scientific and professional knowledge acquired through theory- and research-based principles but altered based on salient aspects of the clinical presentation of the specific patient in light of past clinical experiences.	Discerns when maximum potential and gains from treatment are reached and discharge is appropriate.	Demonstrates exquisite foresight in anticipating developmental needs of patients and self.
Is primarily guided by scientific and professional knowledge acquired through theory and research-based principles.	With guidance, is able to determine patient's maximum potential and gains from treatment.		Critically evaluates own decision-making and judgments.
Recognizes clinical patterns and analyzes and interprets patient's performance to determine differential diagnosis and recommendations.			Develops innovative approaches to care.

ENTRY	CLINICIAN	ADVANCED CLINICIAN	CLINICAL SCHOLAR
With guidance, incorporates acquired theoretical knowledge and research findings to achieve individualized intervention.	Utilizes available community and professional resources to ensure proper intervention throughout the continuum of care.

Considers the relationship among medical diagnosis, symptoms, and reason for referral. | Skillfully analyzes and utilizes available community and professional resources to ensure proper intervention throughout the continuum of care.

Is beginning to take clinical risks not only based on previous clinical experiences but also intuition.

Conducts independent learning based on his/her needs and integrates information into clinical care. | Utilizes a framework for the analyses and interpretation of clinical findings that incorporates the description of human functioning and disability as predictors of outcome.

Utilizes a systematic approach to evaluation and management of patients that is intuitive in their practice, but based on sound theoretical knowledge and clinical experiences.

Utilizes time effectively, fluidly shifting activities and tasks based on patient's performance and reactions to intervention.

Anticipates problems that may arise and implements preventive measures. |

TABLE B.16 Levels of Practice: Speech–Language Pathology—Teamwork and Collaboration

ENTRY	CLINICIAN	ADVANCED CLINICIAN	CLINICAL SCHOLAR
Seeks and values collaborative relationships among support departments.	Provides guidance to less experienced staff.	Acts as a resource to colleagues.	Skillfully negotiates conflict to promote collaboration.
Peer development focuses on learning needs of individual peers.	Identifies improvement related to practice and/or systems.	Recognizes the need for consultation and institutes referrals that will result in mobilization of resources to meet patient and family needs.	Peer development focuses on elevating the standard of practice as a whole.
Contributes to the effective operation of his/her department.	Actively participates in operations-improvement activities.	Promotes the development of collaborative relationships with colleagues by communicating in a constructive manner.	Implements unique and innovative approaches to meeting development needs of self and others.
Identifies the value of operations-improvement activities.	Identifies and values experienced colleagues as an enriching resource to their own practice.		Challenges and shapes the system to maximize the benefits for patient care.
Understands his/her role as an equal member of the healthcare team.	Acknowledges contributions made by colleagues and uses information during own clinical decision-making.	Respects and values contributions of colleagues and acknowledges their work.	Leads/coordinates operations-improvement activities affecting his/her work area and/or patient population.
Seeks and values collaborative relationships with other disciplines to enhance patient management.	Supports colleagues and embraces collaboration by offering and welcoming assistance.	Incorporates joint decision-making into practice.	Achieves credibility; consultation is sought by peers and members of the healthcare team in planning patient care.
Recognizes the value of working in tandem with others to reach mutual goals.		Utilizes conflict resolution skills in response to difficult situations and conflicts with colleagues.	Assimilates pertinent data, communicates to selected team members, and delegates appropriately to achieve desired outcomes.

ENTRY	CLINICIAN	ADVANCED CLINICIAN	CLINICAL SCHOLAR
Recognizes and utilizes resources available to enhance self-professional growth.	Utilizes resources and systems available to enhance patient care and self-professional growth.	Participates in operations-improvement initiatives and evaluates outcomes to determine future goals and activities.	Identifies and utilizes appropriate resources to provide outcome-focused consultation. Promotes growth and creativity of peers and other team members.

© Massachusetts General Hospital

Index of Authors of Clinical Narratives on Interdisciplinary Team Partnerships

Index

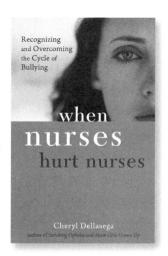
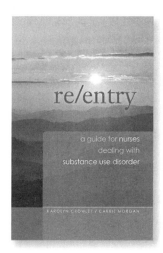
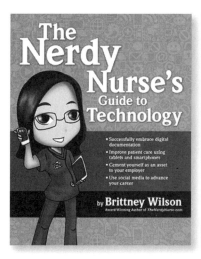
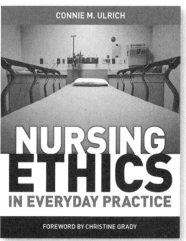

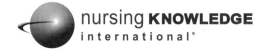

From the Honor Society of Nursing,
Sigma Theta Tau International

The Nurse Manager's Guide Series

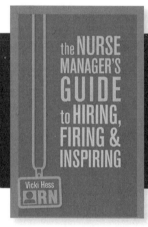

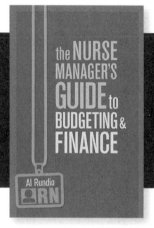

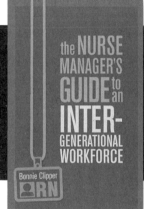

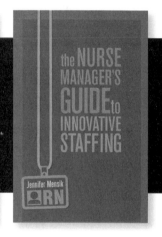

The Nurse Manager's Guide to Hiring, Firing & Inspiring

Vicki Hess

The Nurse Manager's Guide to Budgeting & Finance

Al Rundio

The Nurse Manager's Guide to an Intergenerational Workforce

Bonnie Clipper

The Nurse Manager's Guide to Innovative Staffing

Jennifer Mensik

Sigma Theta Tau International
Honor Society of Nursing®

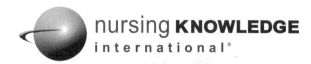